The
Facts
of **Life**
...and More

The
Facts
of Life
...and More

Sexuality and Intimacy for
People with Intellectual
Disabilities

edited by

Leslie Walker-Hirsch, M.Ed., FAAMR
Moonstone
Sexuality Consultation and Education Services
Yorktown Heights, New York
and Santa Fe, New Mexico

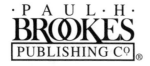
·P·A·U·L·H·
BROOKES
PUBLISHING CO.®

Baltimore • London • Sydney

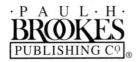

Paul H. Brookes Publishing Co.
Post Office Box 10624
Baltimore, Maryland 21285-0624

www.brookespublishing.com

Typeset by Spearhead Global, Inc., Bear, Delaware.
Manufactured in the United States of America by
Versa Press, Inc., East Peoria, Illinois.

The individuals described in this book are composites or real people whose situations have been masked and are based on the authors' experiences. Names and identifying details have been changed to protect confidentiality.

The photographs that appear throughout the book are used by permission of the individuals pictured or their parents or guardians.

Cover art by Melinda K. Hall.

Library of Congress Cataloging-in-Publication Data

The facts of life—and more : sexuality and intimacy for people with intellectual disabilities / [edited by] Leslie Walker-Hirsch.
    p.   cm.
    Includes index.
    ISBN-13: 978-1-55766-714-4
    ISBN-10: 1-55766-714-4
    1. People with mental disabilities—Sexual behavior. 2. Sex instruction
    for people with mental disabilities. 3. Interpersonal relations.
    4. Intimacy (Psychology) I. Walker-Hirsch, Leslie. II. Title.
HQ30.5F33 2007
306.7087′4—dc22   2006033956

British Library Cataloguing in Publication data are available from the British Library.

Contents

About the Editor

Leslie Walker-Hirsch, M.Ed., FAAMR, President, Social Development and Sexuality Consultant, Moonstone Sexuality Consultation and Education Services, 935 Hanover Street, Yorktown Heights, NY 10598 and 604 Los Altos Norte, Santa Fe, NM 87501

Leslie Walker-Hirsch is the president of Moonstone, a private consultancy and clinical practice specializing in social development, sexuality education, and consultation for individuals with intellectual disabilities, their families, professionals, schools, states, and agencies that support them. She has a master's degree in special education and administration. She is the founder of the American Association on Mental Retardation (AAMR) Special Interest Group on Social and Sexual Concerns, is former President of the AAMR General Division, and serves on the National Clinical Advisory Board of the National Down Syndrome Society. She is a co-creator of the CIRCLES® curriculum series.

About the Contributors

John D. Allen, M.S., Program Director, Employment Services, Marrakech, Inc., 6 Lunar Drive, Woodbridge, CT 06525

John D. Allen is Program Director of Employment Services at Marrakech, Inc., a human services agency based in Woodbridge, Connecticut. Allen is currently a doctoral candidate at Southern Connecticut State University who has a master's degree in urban studies and a bachelor of science in economics. He is the founder of the New Haven Gay & Lesbian Community Center and the Rainbow Support Group. John lives in Branford, Connecticut, with his partner, Keith Hyatte, the Charge Scenic Artist at Long Wharf Theatre.

John J. Barisa, M.A., Psychologist, Psychological Perspectives, 27 Salem Acre, Weaverville, NC 28787

John J. Barisa has dedicated his practice to the treatment and service of individuals with developmental disabilities and coexisting psychiatric conditions. He has developed his own unique methods in treatment, with emphasis on person-centered approaches in all areas, including sexuality. John J. Barisa has developed Psychological Perspectives, a clinic dedicated to service delivery and specific training for clinicians to work with developmental disabilities.

Marklyn P. Champagne, M.S.W., RN, Independent Clinical Social Worker, East Greenwich, RI

Marklyn P. Champagne, a registered nurse and licensed independent clinical social worker, has more than 30 years of expertise in the field of intellectual disabilities. She maintains a private practice in East Greenwich, Rhode Island, for consultation, individual therapy, group education, and creative solutions in issues of social and sexual development for individuals with intellectual disabilities. She is the co-creator of the CIRCLES® curriculum series.

Amy Gerowitz, M.Ed., M.A., M.B.A., President, OUTLOOKS, Cincinnati, OH

Amy Gerowitz is President of OUTLOOKS, a consultation and training firm specializing in organization process improvement, board training, strategic planning and team building for public and private organizations. She was formerly President and Chief Executive Officer of Active Learning Systems, a company that provided central supports for public and private residential agencies. She is a former president of the American Association on Mental Retardation Community Living Division.

Melinda K. Hall, B.B.A, Artist, Santa Fe, NM

Melinda K. Hall is an artist living and working in Santa Fe, New Mexico. She graduated with a bachelor's of business administration from Southern Methodist University in Dallas, Texas and continued her postgraduate studies in fine arts at New Mexico State University. Her work has been seen in gallery and museum venues, as well as in public and private collections, both nationally and internationally since 1990.

Robert Joseph, Ph.D., Sexuality Consultant/Psychologist, New York, NY

Robert Joseph is a licensed New York State psychologist and sexuality consultant. He received his doctorate from the City University of New York. He has 26 years of experience with developmental disabilities, 19 specializing in sexuality and disability. He lives in New York City with his wife and his cat. Robert presents on the topic of disabilities throughout the Northeast.

Emily Perl Kingsley, B.A., Writer, Briarcliff Manor, NY

Emily Perl Kingsley, winner of 16 Emmy Awards and a writer for *SESAME STREET* since 1970, is the mother of an adult with Down syndrome. She was instrumental in integrating children and adults with cognitive and physical disabilities into the format of *SESAME STREET*. She is the author of "Welcome to Holland," an essay that has been reprinted around the world. She has served as a member of the National Media Council on Disability, a group working to improve the ways in which people with disabilities are portrayed in the media. Recently, Ms. Kingsley was appointed to serve on the advisory board for a new partnership formed between *SESAME STREET* and the Special

Olympics. She has also been appointed to the advisory board of the Anti-Defamation League Miller Early Childhood Initiative to combat prejudice and hate.

Ruth Luckasson, J.D., Professor, University of New Mexico, College of Education, Albuquerque, NM 87131

Ruth Luckasson is a Regents' Professor and Professor of Special Education at the University of New Mexico, where she is Chair of the Department of Educational Specialties. She serves on the Board of Trustees of the Judge David L. Bazelon Center for Mental Health Law and The Arc-US Legal Rights and Advocacy Committee. Professor Luckasson is a past president of the American Association on Mental Retardation (AAMR) and has served on the President's Committee on Mental Retardation and as Chair of the American Bar Association's Commission on Mental and Physical Disability Law. Professor Luckasson has published widely on the legal rights of individuals with cognitive disabilities and is co-author of the 9th and 10th editions of *Mental Retardation: Definition, Classification, and Systems of Supports* (AAMR, 1992, 2002).

Stuart A. Lustberg, M.D., FACOG, Obstetrician/Gynecologist, Huntington, NY

Stuart A. Lustberg graduated from the State University of New York at Stony Brook Medical School in 1989 and completed his residency training in Obstetrics and Gynecology at Long Island Jewish Medical Center in1993. He was accepted as a Fellow of the American College of Obstetrics and Gynecology in 1994. He resides with his wife and three children on Long Island in Huntington, New York, where he has maintained a private practice in obstetrics and gynecology since 1993.

Sherry Niccolai, M.A., Educational Diagnostician, Round Rock Independent School District, 1311 Round Rock Avenue, Round Rock, TX 78681

Sherry Niccolai recently graduated with two master's-level degrees: one in Spanish and the other in special education from the University of New Mexico. She is currently working in the Austin Independent School District as a bilingual special education teacher.

Nancy Parello, B.A., Communications Director, Association for Children of New Jersey, 35 Halsey Street, Newark, NJ 07102

Nancy Parello is the Communications Director for the Association for Children of New Jersey, a statewide child advocacy organization. Previously, she worked as a newspaper reporter for 16 years. She lives in Hunterdon County, New Jersey, with her sons, Alex and Ben.

Shay Platz, B.F.A., Photographer, Brooklyn, NY

Shay Platz is currently working in the New York metropolitan area. She is a recent graduate of Rhode Island School of Design with a bachelor of fine arts in photography. She has an interest in portraying people with disabilities in a realistic and sensitive way. For more information visit www.ShayPlatz.com or e-mail Shay@ShayPlatz.com.

Melissa Rennie, B.S., Community News Coordinator, Times Herald Record, Monticello, NY

Melissa Rennie is currently Community News Coordinator for the Sullivan County Bureau of the Times Herald-Record in Monticello, New York. She has written and edited numerous articles on risk management, advocacy, and inclusion related to people with intellectual disabilities. Her work has appeared in publications by the Irwin Siegel Agency and Frontline Initiatives. She is the former associate director of residential programs for Sullivan County ARC. She is a volunteer in several programs serving people with disabling conditions.

John Rose, M.A., Vice President, Irwin Siegel Agency, 25 Lake Louise Marie Road, Rock Hill, NY 12775

John Rose is currently Vice President of the Irwin Siegel Agency, and has a master's degree in public policy. He is the past chairperson of the American Association on Mental Retardation (AAMR) SIG on Direct Support Professionals and received the AAMR Presidential Award for Leadership. He currently serves as a trustee for the American Network of Community Options and Resources Foundation and is also a founding member of the Ontario Association on Developmental Disabilities in Canada.

Mary E. White, M.S., Nurse Practitioner, Dolan Family Health Center, 284 Pulaski Road, Greenlawn, NY 11740

Mary E. White is a women's health care nurse practitioner specializing in family planning, treatment of sexually transmitted diseases, and wellness care of women for over 20 years. She is a nurse colposcopist and has completed a fellowship in HIV/AIDS. She currently provides care to the medically underserved and underinsured at a community health center in Long Island, New York.

Preface

If you are reading this book, *The Facts of Life...and More: Sexuality and Intimacy for People with Intellectual Disabilities,* you are probably either a student, a teacher, a parent, or a professional who wants to develop a better understanding of the complexities associated with sexuality and intellectual disabilities.

You may want to become more knowledgeable about sexuality and intellectual disability because you are taking a course, writing a paper, or have a child, youth or adult offspring, or a student who you see engaged in the process of exploring any part of the lifelong process of social and sexual development.

Whatever your personal reason for embarking upon this reading adventure, I am glad that you are!

A PERSONAL STORY

When I first became an administrator for a small community residential program in New England, I had just enrolled in a master's degree program in special education and administration. Little did I know that these two choices would lead me to become a social development and sexuality educator and advocate for youth and adults with intellectual disability!

My job description as Administrator and Assistant to the Executive Director meant my duties included, among other tasks, interfacing with state and federal funding and oversight agencies, working with health agencies, staff, residents, and the community, as well as "special assignments" as yet undesignated. When someone mentioned the word *sex,* we all either laughed nervously or shuddered or sighed in relief that there were no sexual issues within our programs!

One day a person with an intellectual disability was arrested and accused of inappropriately touching a child. The police, state agency personnel, administrators, and clinicians from our agency were all called together to decide what to do and whether charges would be filed or not. The allegation had been made and could not be ignored, as was the temptation.

The members of our agency knew that this *must* be a misunderstanding by the accusing parents or, in the worst-case scenario, an error in judgment on the part of the resident. The man who was accused was someone we had known for years and who had never been in this kind of difficulty before. We also knew that if this man were to be convicted and end up in the prison system, he would probably not fare very well. Most prisoners with intellectual disabilities do extremely poorly in adapting to prison society! The accusing family wanted this man and all of the residents with intellectual disabilities to leave town.

To our relief a deal was made: Our agency would provide sex education for the accused man as well as for the other individuals with intellectual disabilities to prevent anyone there from making this error again. The committee could evaluate the situation again in a few months time. The director assigned me the job of finding someone to run a sex education class for nine adults with mild intellectual disabilities. It took some time to discover that there was no one out there who had done this before or was interested in doing it now. And so the start of a sexuality education program became one of those previously undesignated items in my job description. After a lengthy telephone conversation with a nurse in the area, we decided to jointly undertake this assignment! And so my involvement with sexuality education of people with cognitive limitations had officially begun. That was in 1979, and I have learned a lot since then!

After more than 25 years of conducting sexuality training classes for youth and adults with disabilities, training countless psychologists, teachers, social workers, administrators, parents, and direct service staff, I feel compelled to record the experiences that I have had and the techniques and strategies that I have developed and used and communicate them to you. Some of these were incorporated into the CIRCLES® curriculum series that I have co-developed with Marklyn P. Champagne. Others I have shared during individual consultation, keynote addresses, training institutes and publications.

Who would have thought that a single incident would become a defining moment, leading me to my calling and my life work in assisting others to undertake sexuality education for individuals with intellectual disabilities! This book is an attempt to share some of those experiences with you.

Because sexuality is a delicate and personal subject, it is difficult to discuss in a candid and meaningful way, even among professionals. The personal stories that are included illustrate some of the range of dimension involved in addressing sexuality issues with individuals with intellectual disabilities.

This book seeks to inform practice. I have written several of these chapters to begin to discuss sexuality and intellectual disability from a social development perspective that is related to age, attitude, culture, family and personal values, scientific and educational knowledge, and beliefs. The chapters incorporate special education techniques and strategies in order to help people with intellectual disabilities access the information and knowledge that every other adult has about adult life. The case stories that I have included dramatize events that have actually happened, although changes and condensations have been made for the sake of confidentiality and space. They will give you insight into the importance that sexuality has in the lives of people with intellectual disability and a window into their thought processes and feelings, their hopes and dreams.

I have invited a number of guest authors who are experts in their respective fields to contribute to this book. These distinguished professionals share my philosophy and prove themselves daily in their practices. I am honored that they have taken time out to communicate to you about their work. You will find that there are extensive references at the end of each chapter. However, this field is still emerging and many of the gifted practitioners contributing to this book used techniques they developed years ago in absence of an adequate field of published knowledge. Only later could they find research to support their techniques and understanding, and in some cases, this research is still missing. The need for knowledgeable professionals in this specialty is one of the reasons this book exists.

When you have finished reading this book, it is my hope and expectation that you will better appreciate the importance of sexuality in all of our lives: for health, for protection, for quality of life, for normalcy, and for personal satisfaction. I also hope that you will be inspired to continue this pioneering work by adding new information and further research to sexuality and intellectual disability.

I expect that you will be a better advocate for the people with intellectual disability that you love, support, teach, and serve and that you will become a force for growth and change in the direction that makes life better for everyone. Please continue reading and enjoy the experience of learning.

Acknowledgments

When I began this project, I really believed that I would simply write down everything I knew about social development and sexuality for individuals with intellectual and developmental disabilities and VOILA! A book would emerge. Little did I know about how many people it takes to REALLY write and produce a work called a book!

Here is a partial list of the people and organizations, in alphabetical order, that I would like to thank:

Marie Abate
Albuquerque Public Schools
Sid Blanchard
Marilyn Bunce
Teddy Bunce
Community Access Unlimited of New Jersey
Marklyn P. Champagne
John Drescher
Sue Drescher
Rita Harris
Debbie Jenkins
Michael Goldstein
Rebecca Lazo
Barbara Levitz
Kathy Marcus
Larry Marcus
Steve Peterson
Christina Ricard
Barry Rosenthal Studio
Cynthia Smalley
The University of New Mexico
James Williams

This book is dedicated to my true loves....

To my darling husband, Bennett Hirsch...
for the joy and delight of his embrace;
for his comfort, encouragement, friendship,
and support

To my spirited, creative,
and always surprising children who I adore:
Jason Wertheimer, Alissa Mazar, and Neal Hirsch...
for growing up to be as they are

To my present and future grandchildren...
for making the world new again

To my friends and colleagues...
for taking time from their hectic lives
to share their brilliance with me

To the children and adults with disabilities
and their families who I have known...
for teaching me how to love

I

Special Education Meets Sexuality Education

1

Sexuality Education and Intellectual Disability Across the Lifespan

A Developmental, Social, and Educational Perspective

Leslie Walker-Hirsch

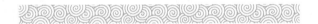

WHAT IS SEXUALITY? WHAT IS SEXUALITY EDUCATION?

The word *sexuality* is an emotionally loaded one! When the word *sexuality* is paired with the similarly emotionally laden term *intellectual disability*, it can engender great discomfort, fear, and uncertainty for parents and professionals, teachers and administrators, and young and old alike.

According to the World Health Organization (WHO), "Sexuality is a central aspect of being human throughout life and encompasses sex, gender identities and roles, sexual orientation, eroticism, pleasure, intimacy and reproduction" (1975). Sexuality is the essence of being a male or female; it is the lens through which a person views the world! There are biological, medical, social, psychological, spiritual, cultural, and legal aspects to sexuality, and these aspects differ depending on where, when, and how you live; who is raising you; and what is personally important to you (WHO, 1975).

When we mention the term *sexuality education*, what image comes to your mind? If you see a balanced set of equations in which

SEXUALITY = HAVING SEX

OR

SEXUALITY EDUCATION = LEARNING TO HAVE SEX

then you need to get a new vision and a new math book! Those are not balanced equations! Sexuality is a much larger topic than just sexual intercourse, and seeing sexuality with limited scope can lead to misunderstanding in how to provide that valuable information to your students.

If you see sexuality education as a yardstick, you might say that only the last inch represents sexual intercourse while the other 35 inches of the yardstick occupy a much larger and more important space. This is a much more realistic image of how we view sexuality education. Consequently, this view affords an increased opportunity to provide meaningful sexuality education to your students that will serve them well throughout their lives. If the image of a yardstick is more like your understanding of sexuality education, then you are on the right track!

If we equate sexuality with having sex, however, we are likely to limit education to sexual intercourse only and ignore the majority of the sexuality education that students need. When we apply a very limited scope to the definition of sexuality education in relation to people with intellectual or developmental disabilities, for example, we mislead their families and teachers into thinking that if a person does not have a sexual partner or does not have the capacity to consent to sexual intercourse, then he or she does not have sexuality and does not need sexuality education at all. Such a limited vision can create fears that sex educators are promoting sexual activity that students are not interested in, that they are not ready for, and that is too great a risk.

The purpose of this book is to provide information to help replace some of the negativity and discomfort that is often associated with sexuality and intellectual disability with optimism, comfort, and normalcy. The chapters in this book will help to answer the following question: How can those who know and care about children, youth, and adults with intellectual disabilities help them to integrate positive, safe, responsible, and legal sexual expression into a high-quality life?

EVERYONE HAS SEXUALITY AND EVERYONE MATURES

Social maturity and sexual development are universal, normal, expected, and inevitable occurrences in the lives of people with or without intellectual disabilities. As with individuals without intellectual disabilities, the timetable for biological maturity for individuals with intellectual disabilities usually coincides with their chronological age (American Academy of Pediatrics, 1996). This is to say the numerical age of onset of physical maturity and puberty for youngsters with intellectual disabilities will be overwhelmingly similar to that for children and youth without intellectual disabilities. The differences in overall maturity between individuals with intellectual disabilities and same-age peers without such disabilities lie in several areas of development beyond just biological maturity, such as social maturity, emotional maturity, educational opportunities, intellectual processing of life experiences, and range of opportunities for real-life learning. Consequently the social, emotional, experiential, and developmental milestones of a young person with an intellectual disability probably will not coincide with the biological ones (Schwier & Hingsburger, 2000). This fact is perhaps the single most important consideration in understanding and successfully implementing sexuality education for students with intellectual disabilities, with social inclusion, sexual safety, and life enjoyment as the primary goals.

THE DEVELOPMENT OF SEXUALITY: UNDERSTANDING THE BIG PICTURE

Genetic sex is determined almost instantly after conception: The genetic sex of the developing cells depends on the genetic material that is contained in a sperm when the sperm meets the egg. The cell cluster will develop as genetically male (XY) if the fertilizing sperm carries a Y chromosome, or it will develop as genetically female (XX) if the fertilizing sperm carries an X chromosome. And so sexual development and sexuality begin, but they continue to be influenced prior to birth (Vandenbergh, 2003).

Before an infant is born, its sexual systems are developed. Male and female organs begin to differentiate from each other during the embryonic stage of development, between 2 and 8 weeks. By the fourth month of development many specific sex organs are identifiable in both male and female fetuses (Vander Zanden, 2000). In addition to sex organ development, some aspects of sexuality are decided before a child is born—aspects over which a parent has had very little control—for example, genetic sex, atypical genetic combinations, delivery complications or injuries, and sensory experiences related to sexual stimulation.

After the birth of the child, environmental, cultural, and social influences come into play to influence sexuality. Some of these influences include

- How the child is carried, nurtured, and cared for
- How the child is dressed, groomed, and toileted
- How the child expects to be touched and handled

- How long the child is allowed to cry
- The kinds of toys and stimulation that the child enjoys and receives
- How the rest of the world interacts with the child as either a boy or a girl

As you can see, many important lessons of a child's sexuality education are taught long before puberty. Parents and family members are the first, most influential and most important sex educators of young children. How parents regard each other and their children and how parents teach their children to enjoy and regard their bodies are important parts of early sexuality education. And the expectations and interactions parents and their children have with others in their social world all contribute as well.

Environmental events and cultural practices at a particular time in history influence the interpretation of masculinity or femininity in particular cultures. For example, wearing trousers or slacks was considered to be a masculine form of dress. Today it is acceptable for both males and females to wear slacks and wearing slacks is no longer considered an expression of masculinity. In addition, many occupations that have traditionally been held by women, such as nurse or secretary, now include many more men. The reverse is also true; women now pursue traditionally male occupations like firefighter, soldier, electrician, or scientist. As a child's awareness grows, family social practices interact with the personal characteristics of the child in even more noticeable ways. Children frequently replicate family routines and practices (Mattis, 1994).

The following list includes some of the many factors that influence social and sexual expectations that are in action long before a child enters school, and way, way before puberty appears on the horizon:

- How family members give and receive affection to and from the child and each other
- How privacy and modesty are expressed at home
- How family members demonstrate and communicate being happy, sad, angry, or afraid, as well as more subtle emotional messages
- How family members argue and make up from arguments
- How family members interact with friends and social contacts outside of the family
- How family members interact with authority figures
- How family members teach each other (Couwenhoven, 2001)

A child with an intellectual disability that includes autism or autistic-like behaviors may have significant limitations in the ability to replicate his or her parents' social behaviors and the ability to understand social interactions, even with close family members.

The presence of an intellectual disability and the experiences a child with an intellectual disability has may affect his or her self-perception and the family's perception of that child as being nonsexual or as being younger than his or her chronological age and biological maturity indicate.

For example, the nature of some disabilities requires intense medical procedures (e.g., surgery, physical therapy) over the course of many years. These invasive procedures may lead to physical and emotional reactions that can affect a child's subsequent understanding and interpretation of social and sexual boundaries. Even difficult toilet training or prolonged toileting assistance may color a child's social expectations as he or she continues to mature (Melby, 2001).

Parents must make judgments about family routines that serve their child's interest and must also decide the right time to implement any needed changes in those routines that address the needs of their child with a disability as well as the needs of other family members. Modesty and privacy of all of the family members can be integrated into daily household activities and considered ordinary, but they are important aspects of early sexuality education.

Sam is a charming child with Down syndrome, who has a sister, Barbara, who is two years older than him. Sam has a penchant for both the humorous and the dramatic! Starting when he was 4 years old Sam loved to take a bath in the evening and then run naked through the house to find his father and jump into his lap. He would get his nightly tickle from his dad and then run to get ready for bed. This was fun for everyone! Sam continued this routine for many years, but when he turned 12, he began to physically mature. His naked antics every night were no longer appropriate, especially with his 14-year-old sister present and sometimes her friends as well. Sam's parents did not realize that even if they themselves did not find a physically mature child being unclothed to be a problem in their own household, that Barbara's friends and their parents would probably find it objectionable. Barbara's friends were not allowed to visit in the evening or sleep over.

Sam's parents realized that punishment and loss of privilege were not the answer to breaking this routine. Positively influencing Sam to change his behavior, however, required a bit of ingenuity. For his 13th birthday, his parents gave him several sets of superhero pajamas and slippers. Each night he chose which costume he wanted to take into the bathroom for the after-bath "Superhero Olympics." Sam got to choose his outfit and a laughter-filled tumble with Dad continued to follow bath time but with attention to modesty. This change allowed for a more adult atmosphere that was more comfortable for Sam's parents and for his sister Barbara and her friends.

SOCIAL DEVELOPMENT

Sexuality education at home does not usually come in the form of a formal class or an easily identified lesson. It is usually established through training and the promotion of acceptable behaviors that consider the many elements of a busy household.

When a child with a disability enters a school program nowadays, he or she will, in all likelihood, enter an inclusive setting. This means that a child with a disability will have the opportunity to play with, learn with, and befriend same-age peers who may be more developed in social, emotional, and experiential ways. This also may be the first time that the child is out of his or her parents' sight for long periods of time. Suddenly, this child has experiences unseen by the parents and often unreported to them by their child, especially if there is low language or communication development. When children enter school, they experience new friends, opportunities, learning styles, routines, authorities, cultures, and roles. This is as true for parents as it is for their children.

Most children with and without disabilities benefit socially from an inclusive classroom experience. In the elementary grades, for example, friendships between children with and without disabilities can develop at storytime, during recess, at the painting easel, in the Boy and Girl Scouts, and at birthday parties.

Typically developing children between the ages of 5 and 8 years are curious about many things and are not usually inhibited about asking questions about sexual matters. Providing information gradually to children at this age is an excellent way to provide a foundation for later discussions about more complex and adult sexual matters. Discussions with children of this age may include the development of new family routines of privacy and modesty as well as an opportunity to ease fears that arise over partial understanding of nonfiction news or stories about, for example, HIV/AIDS or fictional entertainment about sex and violence (Mattis, 1994).

Children with intellectual or developmental disabilities may demonstrate these same characteristics, sometimes beginning at a later chronological age and continuing even into adolescence or later if there are very significant developmental delays. It can become more complicated when the child with a disability is mature in appearance but immature in social development. Despite a child's developmental maturity, communities often expect the child to conform to the sexual norms of behavior primarily based upon the age the child *looks* (American Academy of Pediatrics, 1996). This means that public displays of affection, personal modesty, use of privacy, recognizing private sexual body areas and associated acceptable behaviors, and differentiating private localities from public ones are the focus of sexuality education for many of the preadolescent years.

Masturbation, or the touching of genitals as a way of experiencing a pleasurable feeling, is a widely observed activity in infancy. Many children will discover the pleasurable sensation of masturbation during middle childhood if they did not discover it during infancy. Although children do not have erotic fantasies, sexual pleasure and intention is likely to be present during masturbation, although relaxation and stress relief are also acknowledged benefits. Sexuality education about genital stimulation at this age should focus on when and where masturbation is acceptable without social stigma, rather than on instilling shame or guilt about the enjoyment of the act itself (Planned Parenthood Federation of America & American Association of Sex Educators, Counselors, and Therapists, 2003).

Many parents report that their children or older adolescents masturbate as a way to fill time when boredom, loneliness, or a lack of complex recreation skills or opportunities are observed to be present, perhaps as precipitating factors. According to Planned Parenthood, 70% percent of men in their twenties and 50% of women in their thirties masturbate. Genital stimulation while alone and in private is thought to be a rehearsal for mature adult sex play, but it also is a vehicle for pleasure and fulfillment at a mature age (Planned Parenthood Federation of America & American Association of Sex Educators, Counselors, and Therapists, 2003).

Masturbation among mature adolescents with intellectual disabilities must conform to the social standards that the law and community set for other adults. When frequent masturbation interferes with participation in other social outlets and stimulating activities, family members or school staff should consult an expert in sexuality for those with intellectual or developmental disabilities and their families to provide evaluation and guidance about how to proceed in either education, environmental changes, behavior therapy, counseling, or sex therapy.

Family and cultural traditions and beliefs are also factors in what education and structure about masturbation a family desires to provide. For example, clinicians and religious scholars can interpret the meaning of the biblical reference to the sin of Onan as a punishment for failure to provide an heir rather than as a prohibition against masturbation itself (Planned Parenthood Federation of America & American Association of Sex Educators, Counselors, and Therapists, 2003).

CHILDHOOD FRIENDSHIPS

Around the time of approaching puberty, there is often a change in childhood friendships. Many developing teens have their own struggle with the changes that puberty is imposing upon them. Typically developing teens often manage the feelings that accompany the changes of puberty with conformity: same sneakers, same hairdos, same movie and music idols, and the extreme importance of being accepted by their peers. They may be less able to manage the added stress that having a friend who may be atypical can bring to bear. In contrast, young people with intellectual disabilities are less likely to know the subtleties of conforming to the latest teenage dress code or music innovation. This "out of step" look can further isolate a child with an intellectual disability from the flow of teenage events. Rejection by previously treasured friends appears to be a frequent, sad, and misunderstood occurrence.

Parents' concern for safety can also add to the developmental rift that often happens at this time. The degree of independence that typically developing preteens or teens are given by their parents is usually greater than the degree of independence parents of preteens with intellectual disabilities feel is appropriate for their children. This limits some of the social opportunities that bond friends together at this time, such as going to the mall without parental supervision, e-mailing and instant messaging friends, or independently attending a movie. These are teenage social experiences that may not be within safe or easy reach of preteens or teens with disabilities. As a result of such social isolation, preteens or teens with intellectual disabilities may become estranged from the friendships of an earlier time.

> Marlena is 13 years old and has a mild intellectual disability. She has several friends that she has known since elementary school. One day her friends, Alice and Kathy, were going to the mall with Alice's mother. Marlena was invited to go, too. Marlena was excited and delighted. They picked Marlena up and went to the mall. The three girls went to look at CDs while Alice's mother went to buy shoes next door. When Alice's mother returned to find the girls, Marlena was not with them. Alice explained that Marlena decided she had to use the bathroom and left to go there. The security guards found Marlena unharmed at the other end of the mall. Alice's mother never invited Marlena to go with them again because she could not manage the responsibility of keeping track of Marlena or trusting her to stay with the other girls.

In addition, the intellectual accomplishments and interests of typically developing teens can be of a more adult nature than those of teens with cognitive delays.

Jamal is 15 years old and has a moderate developmental disability. He has a brother who is one year younger than he is. Jamal was frequently invited to spend time with his brother's friends when they went to school activities or played video games. They have also invited him to hang out with them without a structured agenda or planned activity. On one such occasion, the friends were interested in talking about girls and watching baseball. Jamal, however, could not follow the baseball game and did not have interest in or permission to go on dates. He wanted to watch the Cartoon Network and make animal noises as each different animal character came on, but he did not have a friend who would also think that was a fun way to spend the afternoon. After an hour or so, Jamal began to behave in a very silly, then in a loud, then in an aggressive way toward his brother's friends, who had tried to include him in their leisure pursuits.

After this happened several times, Jamal was less welcome to join in with his brother's social activities. He needed friends who liked the same things that he liked, friends who had the same interests he had, friends who wanted to watch the same TV programs and enjoy them in the same way that he enjoyed them.

Even typically developing preteens who are able to maintain friendships with peers with intellectual disabilities that began in elementary school have been observed to change the nature of the friendship from a peer-to-peer friendship to a helping friendship (Staub, 1998).

Jonathan and Kyle grew up on the same street and were born in the same year. Kyle has an intellectual disability and Jonathan does not. Their mothers were frequent companions, and the two boys were friends throughout their elementary school years. Kyle and Jonathan rode the school bus together, ran around the back yard together, and belonged to the same Boy Scout group. These friends sought out each other's company. During Boy Scout meetings, it became clear that Jonathan spent most of his time helping Kyle complete his projects as soon as he finished his own. He also began to intercede when other scouts could not understand Kyle's speech. Jonathan helped Kyle decide which project to do next and how to do it, where to sit at the meetings, and which color to paint his weekly creations. When Jonathan began answering for Kyle, the scoutmaster stopped addressing his questions to Kyle. Instead he asked Jonathan. Little by little, Kyle became dependent on Jonathan to anticipate his needs, and he became passive in his social relationships.

The boys continued to be friends, but their friendship became less of a peer-to-peer relationship and more of a hierarchical, caregiving relationship. This kind of relationship has its benefits, but it is not a replacement for a peer-to-peer friendship.

It is especially important for teachers and family members not to inadvertently devalue friendships that their children with disabilities have with other children with disabilities by overvaluing their friendships with typically developing same-age peers. Some parents may brag to their friends or relatives that their children have only typically developing friends. Some parents may even condone statements by their child that it is acceptable to be afraid of students who have disabilities. By the same token, praising certain individuals for their academic accomplishments or their driving ability may convey an unspoken message about the greater desirability of having friends who do not have disabilities. There is room in a person's life for many different kinds of friends, each with valuable assets to offer. Most of us choose to have relationships with people from many diverse cultures and practices to enjoy and learn from. However, we also align ourselves with friends who evidence a common identity. For example, friendships might develop from common extracurricular interests (e.g., church, ice skating), neighborhood interests and experiences, or similar personal experiences (e.g., new mothers, empty nesters). Relationships often develop in a natural and intuitive way by participation in mutual interests or working side-by-side over a period of time.

When it is time to establish more adult relationships, men and women with intellectual disabilities often will find the greatest likelihood for a satisfactory relationship with another person who has had similar experiences and looks to form a lifestyle with a similar degree of independence and complexity. An adult with an intellectual disability will be expected to live with one foot in the world of disability affiliations and friendships and the other foot in the world that includes broader aspects of society. A prejudice against having relationships with people with intellectual or other disabilities can lead to a boycott of activities that are developed for people with disabilities, such as the Special Olympics, after-school special recreation programs, socialization groups, or life skills courses. This can lead to a lonely life and an extremely limited opportunity for safe, mutual, and reciprocated social interactions and age-appropriate sexual expression. Romance is more likely to be safe and have a more balanced power structure when both participants have similar abilities to negotiate and prevail within the relationship.

Bernard is an adult with a moderate intellectual disability. He lives with his mother and father. He has an adult sister who also lives nearby. Bernard spends all of his nonwork time with his mother and father and their friends and sometimes their family members. He does not participate in any social programs nor does he have any friends.

Bernard had a job in a diner but was fired because he was socially inappropriate and "overly friendly in a sexualized manner" with the other diner employees. Although he was cautioned many times to stop these behaviors, he persisted in them until he was dismissed for sexual harassment. His family stressed that he did not know any better because he had never had any school classes or friends to teach him how to socialize in a more appropriate and mature way. He did not recognize that his co-workers were not his friends. Although his family did not mind repeatedly telling him to stop any unwanted behavior, this characteristic (especially with sexual implications) was not tolerated in a work setting.

PUBERTY ARRIVES ON TIME

At the time of puberty, there are more dramatic events that draw attention to sexual development. Most adolescents with intellectual disabilities show the biological signs of maturity within the typical age range of their peers without disabilities. In an article titled "Yesterday's Precocious Puberty is Norm Today," Jane Brody, Health Editor of *The New York Times,* discussed another article that appeared in the October 4, 1999, issue of the journal *Pediatrics,* in which Drs. P. Kaplowitz, S. Oberfield, and other members of the Lawson Wilkins Pediatric Endocrine Society concluded that in today's time, girls' puberty often begins between the ages of 6 and 8, slowly of course, and in ways that sometimes go unnoticed until later. Brody described this new data as reflecting puberty signs at least one year earlier for girls than was concluded by Dr. Marcia E. Herman-Giddens and colleagues from a study 2 years earlier (Brody, 1999).

That is, somewhere between the ages of 9 and 16, physical maturity becomes evident: Adolescents undergo the growth of body hair, voice changes, breast enlargements, growth spurts, and an intensity of mood that signals adult hormones. However, the gap between physical maturity and social, intellectual, and emotional maturity often begins to widen at this time for teens with developmental or intellectual disabilities. For this reason, additional attention and time needs to be devoted to learning many new behaviors and meeting the more adult expectations that are now necessary.

Many children like to have the spotlight of attention. They can accomplish this honor by being helpful at the grocery store and receiving praise from a high-profile adult or by learning to sing, dance, paint, play an instrument, or in countless other ways. Children who do not get enough attention through positive venues will seek attention in negative ways. When those communications are ignored, children may turn to inappropriate sexual activity as a means to get attention. Children will sometimes go to great lengths not to have their needs for attention ignored, even if it means that they will be reprimanded! A child might pull down his or her pants publicly, make a sexually inappropriate state-ment, or touch him- or herself or others in sexual areas of the body, usu-ally in the genitals or breasts. Schools and families can accept or overlook a great many undesirable behaviors, but inappropriate or dan-gerous sexual behavior gets everyone's attention immediately.

Carl is a high school student with an intellectual disability. Carl was in a high school program that did not meet his needs for socialization. A school aide continuously supervised him, and his academic needs were being met with one-to-one instruction, but there was no opportunity to interact with other students. When academic work got difficult and Carl felt frustrated, he would ask to go to the bathroom. He was never denied, even though his aide knew it was a way to take a break from the frustration of his academic work. Carl's aide would escort him to the bathroom, but she could not accompany him inside. Carl would spend a minute or so in the boys' room and then return to his schoolwork. There was never a problem.

One day, Carl visited a new program that would offer him more social interaction, but he was warned that he needed to have excellent behav-ior or he would not be accepted into the program. Carl was nervous that he would not be accepted into the program. He voiced his reluctance about going to the new program, even for the day, to his parents, but his pleas were ignored. After a few minutes of attending the new school's pro-gram, he said he had to go to the bathroom. An aide escorted him to the bathroom area. Instead of going into the boys' bathroom, Carl went into the girls' bathroom.

School staff members summoned Carl's parents and said that he was too immature to manage the demands of the new program. Carl's parents wanted him to have the advantages that the new program would offer, but they did not want him getting in trouble and getting a bad reputation in the new setting. In the end, Carl's parents did not send him to the new program. They eventually paid attention to Carl's need for security and socialization.

FORMAL SEXUALITY EDUCATION IN SCHOOL

Many children with intellectual disabilities receive formalized sexuali-ty education in mainstream/inclusive health education classes. Often, however, the pace of instruction and the emphasis of the discussions are not effectively oriented to meet the needs of students with cogni-tive disabilities. The idiosyncratic learning styles of special education students often require special educational techniques that support understanding and include extra practice and skill building. For exam-ple, dating may be a topic that is addressed in an inclusive health education course in a high school. Topics are likely to include why a person goes on a date, how a person decides if he or she wants to go or not, how to accept or decline a date, what constitutes safe dating, and how to set sexual limits.

These topics certainly would benefit students with intellectual disabilities. However, students with intellectual disabilities are less likely than their typically developing peers to already have the language, judgment, social/emotional maturity, and adaptive social skills of friendship and negotiation that they can readily generalize to this more adult relationship. Consequently, education about dating for students with intellectual disabilities needs to include numerous opportunities to develop specific language, role playing opportunities as rehearsal, numerous chances to practice asking for a date in a supportive environment, and support in planning the activity and logistics for the date. Often these plans must include parents or other support personnel, and how to approach them, since parents frequently need to provide transportation and even supervision for their teens and adults with intellectual disabilities on a date.

Since it can be embarrassing to practice and receive instruction in this area in an inclusive setting, it may be more practical and of greater benefit to provide this kind of additional training time in a setting that is more private and that can better address the specific needs of the individuals involved. The amount of time needed for a student to become sufficiently capable may interfere with the volume of material that needs to be covered by the health teacher in an inclusive class. The pace of learning that includes rehearsal, practice, and added supports for language and behavior should be at a slower speed to allow the students to practice these specialized techniques. It is possible that supportive teaching strategies may not be used by health education teachers in junior or senior high schools because of time constraints or because the rest of the class is ready for new material and does not require the degree of skill building and repetition necessary for students with intellectual disabilities.

Participation in an inclusive health education class can be supplemented with additional learning time, either during school hours or even in after-school sessions or tutorials, to allow students with intellectual disabilities to benefit from the class discussions and also have a safe setting for role play and rehearsals.

The dilemma of offering comprehensive, age- and ability-appropriate social/sexual education in an inclusive classroom setting becomes quite obvious. It is very important for teens with or without disabilities to have sexuality education that is meaningful and that proceeds in a way that suits their individual experiences and learning capacities. It is often advisable to create smaller groups of adolescents with similar learning capacities to be certain that the sexuality educational content is conveyed in an effective manner and addresses and emphasizes the aspects that are most pressing for each group (Eshilian et al., 2000).

Many of the social skills that are important for assertiveness, expression of feelings, or decision making can be learned in classes other than "sex ed.," even though they are "sex ed. skills." For example, speech and language classes that use conversation partners can arrange to coordinate expressive and receptive language around the topics of friendships and relationships. Specific conversations might include making plans for an after-school activity, expressing preferences, negotiating conflicts, and discussing teen culture. The complexity and the degree of student participation will give teachers an idea about whether the students are "getting it" or simply acquiescing and looking involved.

> Corrinne is a teenager who has been included in her high school program, including health education/sexuality education. Soon after the current term began, Corrinne began to have sleepless nights and had difficulty getting up in the mornings. She began missing the school bus because of morning stomach cramps. Then, one morning she was found under her bed, hysterically crying and very frightened. After some comforting and counseling, her parents discovered that Corrinne's health class was studying teenage health behaviors. What Corrinne took away from the teacher's lessons was: teenagers drink alcohol, do illegal drugs, have sex, and make unwanted babies. She was afraid to go to school with teenagers.

Teens and young adults may have difficulty understanding their disabilities and the ramifications of them in terms of limitations on their independence and their very real need for added safeguards and clinical supports. Denial of the disability is common, especially by the most capable of individuals. Parents frequently report that their children with disabilities demonstrate disability prejudice, which can be manifested by refusal to go to social programs geared for young adults with similar or more obvious disabilities. It can also translate into statements such as, " I want to go out with a girl without any disability," or, "I hate Down syndrome." Long evenings and weekends without companionship can often lead to loneliness, social isolation, boredom, and even depression and desperation. Children and adults with disabilities are most likely to feel the keen edge of exclusion because they have the awareness of the social stigma and rejection that may be attached to their disabilities.

Clarence is a high school student with Down syndrome. He is included in a full academic program, and with hard work and tutoring, he is doing well academically. He is, however, the only included student in his small high school. He has no friends and is not very happy. One afternoon, a small group of "cool" high school boys told Clarence that if he wanted to have lunch with them, he had to prove he was worthy. To be worthy Clarence had to do two things: touch the breasts of the captain of the cheerleading squad and then pull the fire alarm.

Clarence would do anything to have lunch with these guys, even things he knows are wrong and would surely lead him into trouble. Needless to say, Clarence did what the other students wanted him to do in the hopes of having lunch with the guys! Unfortunately, because of his actions, he was suspended from classes and lost privileges at home from his family. He never got to have the highly desired lunch with his supposed friends, and worse, he was the butt of even more jeering at school, leading him to become even more isolated and self-loathing.

PARENTS CONTINUE TO BE SEXUALITY EDUCATORS

Although many aspects of sexuality are either already determined or influenced by forces outside of the safe family environment, parents and siblings continue to fill an important role in providing sexuality education for children with intellectual disabilities. Family members may be considered the reliable and safe sources for accurate information, provided that they also continue to be "askable" authority figures. That is, they do not get angry or frightened or immediately call for a therapist or social worker *and* they are willing to speak frankly about sexuality. This means that if a parent does not know the answer to a question, he or she gets the answer and shares it with the child in a way that is appropriate to the child's age and abilities. It also means that a parent needs to be sensitive enough to ask a questioning teen or young child, "Why are you asking that question?" or "Where did you hear that word?" or "Were you discussing that with someone?" Often this will lead to disclosure of the circumstances leading to the specific question. Disclosures might be related to something that the child heard on the news or perhaps there is a new baby in the family next door and that parent has used some new sexual terms that have stimulated some curiosity or need for verification. Or, in a more sinister event, the disclosure may reveal that the child has experienced or witnessed inappropriate touching. Knowing what precipitates a child's question can guide parents as to how best to answer that question: with reassurance, with facts, with advice, or with pride that they can be the source of personal growth for their child. In this way a parent creates confidence in their child, which helps the child to be able to ask other adult questions and get supportive responses from his or her most trusted adult.

Millie is a 12-year-old pre-teen with a mild intellectual disability. Each night before she goes to bed, she kisses each family member on the cheek to say goodnight. On one night, instead of a peck on the cheek, Millie gave her mother a passionate French kiss! While Millie's mother was both embarrassed and stunned, she addressed the situation calmly. Instead of yelling at her daughter or acting alarmed, Millie's mom asked, "That's not how we usually kiss goodnight in our family. Where did you learn about that kind of kissing?" Millie was proud when she said, "My friend Sheila told me that kissing with your tongue and an open mouth is the *real* way to kiss and that you were afraid to tell me that I was kissing you wrong all these years. She said I should be mad at you for not telling me the truth!" A productive discussion followed about different ways that people kiss, and Millie's mom reassured her that a kiss on the cheek was the exact best way to kiss her family members goodnight. Millie's mom gave her some more adult information about why adults sometimes kissed in a more romantic and passionate way if they had that kind of relationship.

Millie's mom took it one step further and asked if she could speak to Sheila's mother about the different kinds of kissing so that Sheila could have some accurate, new information from her own mother, too. Millie agreed that that was a good idea!

She kissed her mom on the cheek, said goodnight, and went to bed a little later than they planned but with a smile on her face. Millie's mother smiled, too.

THE MEDIA AND SEXUALITY

Many of today's television programs, movies, music, and music videos make references to adult situations and use sexual language. They frequently contain unspoken assumptions about sexual relationships, misunderstandings between the sexes, or jealousy over romantic rivals. These and other widely viewed media programs and movies use sexual innuendo as a source of comic quips. AIDS and HIV are everyday topics on nightly newscasts. Voluptuous female stars often are the draw in movies. Movies, television shows, and magazine advertisements for cars, shampoos, deodorants, perfumes, soft drinks, and beer frequently feature a sales pitch coupled with sexy men and women, which carries an underlying message that these products will enhance the consumer's sex appeal. Stand-up comics spar with their audience by using sexual insults and slang to make a statement and command attention with explicit, and sometimes shocking, sexual vocabulary. Teens and young adults with intellectual disabilities may not understand the meaning of these sexual references, and they may take away that violence or comedy concerns sex, is about people similar to themselves, and that sex is always embarrassing or scary.

Parents can use these media opportunities to discover what their children understand and to help their children to progress toward greater social skill and sophistication. A teachable moment that results from the media's use of sexual subject matter can lead to a good discussion about negotiating relationships, anger management, values, ulterior motives, and errors in judgment. If it is followed by a "Did that ever happen to you?" question, parents can often learn much about the part of the teen's life that happens when parents are not around.

It is exciting that children and youth with intellectual disabilities, like their typically developing peers, can use their computers to communicate with their friends and relatives, surf the web, do homework, play games, improve academic skills, and get information. The Internet, e-mail, and computer e-friends, however, have also added a new set of sexual risks in recent times. The number of sexual solicitations in chat rooms is alarming, and even naïve searches can unwittingly invite pernicious, sexually explicit, or deviant websites to appear on unprotected computer screens. Parental monitoring of e-mails, the installation of lockout systems to prevent unwanted sex and violence from appearing on computers in the home for certain users, and discussion of computer-related experiences can go a long way to making computer activity safer for vulnerable youth and adults with intellectual limitations.

Although there are many, many Internet sites for gaining accurate information about sexuality available for professionals, teachers, parents, and typically developing teens, it is difficult to verify reliable sources on sexuality that are specifically designed for individuals with intellectual disabilities to access independently. Almost any reliable site can provide information that parents and their children with intellectual disabilities can access together.

REDUCING THE RISKS ASSOCIATED WITH SEXUAL VULNERABILITY

Teens and young adults who have intellectual disabilities and who are without adequate sexuality education, have few or no friends, and have little social support are more vulnerable to sexual exploitation. In an attempt to gain social acceptance or to avoid loneliness, individuals with intellectual disabilities are more likely to be manipulated into sexual situations that take advantage of their disabilities and isolation, even placing them at risk of unwanted pregnancy, sexual assault, HIV/AIDS, or other sexually transmitted diseases.

While there are many reasons why individuals with intellectual disabilities are at greater risk, the following risk-reducing, educational interventions may help to counter some of those reasons:

- Develop meaningful sexuality education programs
- Change public perception of people with intellectual disabilities
- Improve or develop social and emotional supports
- Reward and memorialize successes
- Prepare for situations that are unfamiliar
- Counter disability prejudice
- Prevent social isolation and boredom
- Decrease dependence on others for personal care

Develop Meaningful Sexuality Education Programs

Providing meaningful, comprehensive sexuality education is the antidote to vulnerability caused by ignorance. Sometimes a person with an intellectual disability may not even have enough information to know that he or she is being taken advantage of: The person may be told, for example, that "everyone does this with their neighbors." The person may be led to believe that if he or she performs sexual activities and keeps the relationship a secret from family members, the perpetrator will love him or her. Often, individuals with intellectual disabilities who have not received sexuality education do not know that they can refuse sexual advances from anyone, even authority figures such as teachers, family members, or clergy, or can at least report them.

Compliance with the requests of authority figures has often been the rule for behavior that well-meaning parents and teachers have instilled in individuals with intellectual disabilities. There are times when a person with an intellectual disability may know that he or she is engaging in an unwanted sexual activity, but that person may not know how to get help in a situation that is beyond his or her ability to manage. For instance, the person may not be able to dial the phone, may not have the language skills to describe what is happening, or may not know how to take a bus to a rape crisis center.

When these risk factors are present, there is an increased likelihood of vulnerability to sexual abuse for people with intellectual disabilities. Individuals with intellectual disabilities have a significantly higher rate of sexual abuse than same-age peers in the general population (Baladerian, 2003; Sobsey, 1994).

Meaningful sexuality education for individuals with intellectual disabilities can empower many people to both recognize and report sexual abuse. If they are knowledgeable, they are more likely to be taken seriously and to be believed when they make a report.

Change Public Perception of People with Intellectual Disabilities

People with intellectual disabilities are frequently targeted for sexual abuse because they often are perceived as not likely to be good reporters of abuse and less capable of exerting their own power. They are portrayed in the media as being easily manipulated and controlled and less likely to be believed if they do report abuse. They may even be deemed incapable of testifying in court in their own behalf. A comprehensive sexuality education for this group will empower many people to both recognize and report sexual abuse. If they are knowledgeable, they are more likely to be taken seriously and to be believed when they make a report. Comprehensive sexuality education is needed for the general community as well to change their perceptions about the capabilities and resources that are available to people with intellectual disabilities who have had the advantage of meaningful sexuality education.

Improve or Develop Social and Emotional Supports

It is never too late to develop or increase the level of social and emotional support for individuals with intellectual disabilities. Helping a person to understand the value of friendship and practice having and being a friend is an important aspect of social development and sexuality education. Access to friends in an environment where trust in an adult authority figure is available can be a goal of counseling. There are funded resources for youth and adults with intellectual disabilities through community colleges; county mental health centers; local disability services groups, such as The Arc and the local Down Syndrome Society affiliates group; special recreation departments; or other service providers. Counselors associated with a service provider agency usually have access to phone numbers and contact information for local organizations. While a loving family is of course an important aspect of social and emotional support, it is not a substitute for friendships with chosen peers.

Reward and Memorialize Successes

It is true that people with intellectual disabilities often have rejections and failures in forming relationships and in other aspects of nonacademic life. However, they also have successes. These successes can be memorialized and remembered in photos, awards, newsletters, and personal diaries. Being told " Good job!" is not as good as accomplishing a good job and recognizing the feeling of being successful. When an award representing achievement or a photo of a successful experience is viewed, not only is the experience recalled, but also is the feeling of accomplishment. Each success sets the stage for the next and can provide the courage necessary to try again after a setback. However, some parents encourage their children to be content with the level of achievement that they currently have and even hope that their children will avoid new challenges, for fear that the new challenges may result in failure, rather than a goal not attempted.

Prepare for Situations that Are Unfamiliar

Anticipating new behaviors that are likely to be required in new situations can take a great deal of stress out of new situations. Successfully practicing skills can offer the confidence that familiarity can give a person. Here are a few examples:

- A person who is going to a banquet but has only been to fast food restaurants in the past may benefit from rehearsing the social behaviors that are expected there. Rehearsal can ease the tension and anxiety and may reduce the likelihood of being the object of ridicule or trying to get negative attention.

- The first time a young woman gets a gynecological exam, it is important that she knows what to expect. She may need reassurance that it is OK for a medical person to touch her in that way, even if she does not know the person. Distinguishing this touch from a sexual touch may also be in order.

- A young man going to the movies with a date needs to be instructed in the limits of romantic touching that are acceptable in a movie theater.

The effect of receiving accurate information from a trusted authority figure sets the stage for calming anxiety and having better emotional control. Rehearsals and role play of novel or unfamiliar experiences give parameters for recognizing the behavior of others that might overstep the accepted rules for touch, talk, or trust. This reduces vulnerability by increasing the likelihood of reporting variance from the rehearsed scenario.

Counter Disability Prejudice

Disability prejudice can overvalue the friendship offering of a person without a disability. Wanting to be accepted by people without disabilities can lead to sexual compliance by individuals with intellectual disabilities to gain acceptance or praise. The promise of acceptance into a nondisabled social group, event, or activity is a frequent ploy used by sexual predators. It can be an enticement into sexual contact that a person with an intellectual disability may tolerate in order to be included in a desirable activity as a promised reward.

Disability prejudice can also translate into self-hatred. Helping a person recognize that he or she is many things—a woman or man, an athlete, a school member, a knitter, a charity volunteer, a friend, a person with blue eyes—in addition to being a person with a disability, can dissipate the negative power that the disability may hold over the person's evaluation of his or her own worth.

Prevent Social Isolation and Boredom

The confidence that comes from being part of something larger than oneself is a strong opposition to the loneliness that social isolation and boredom offers. An individual who is desperate for friends may tolerate an abusive relationship because it can be perceived as being better than nothing. Learning how to get a friend and be a friend, even in a parallel play activity, reduces the depressing feelings of exclusion and isolation. Many individuals with intellectual disabilities have a more limited number of social contacts and experiences from which to draw: A stimulating and full life that includes safe opportunities to perfect the social skills of friendship, dating, and romance in a nonjudgmental setting may increase the number of opportunities that are available to participate in the larger world. Confidence comes with proven skill.

Direct instruction in the skills of friendship as part of general classroom instruction is important. Receiving recognition when those skills are demonstrated on a daily basis is equally important. Share, care, cooperate, help, and support are five basic learning activities that teachers can teach, notice, praise, and reward among peers. James Stanfield Company and Young Adult Institute (YAI) have video curricula that provide stimulating action videos that demonstrate friendship skills and offer suggestions for follow up and enhancement of skills and behaviors through practice and understanding (*Being With People Video Series*, 1990; YAI, 1993).

Decrease Dependence on Others for Personal Care

People with intellectual disabilities typically need some degree of support with decision making, finances, personal care, health maintenance, and social planning. Some individuals will be more independent than others but are still likely to require some reliance on the good character and intentions of an ever changing array of caregivers. This dependence creates a very complicated relationship when a caregiver becomes sexually abusive. Reporting a violation, if the person is intellectually and physically able to do so, belies the complexity. An authority figure who abuses may also be providing support, sustenance, gifts, transportation, companionship, medical care, and relief from loneliness and boredom to the person with an intellectual disability. While reporting the abuse may put an end to the abuse, it most likely will also cause a loss of the other benefits that the abuser had provided. This creates a very complex set of emotional dynamics.

Nationwide computer registries and networks for identifying prospective personal care assistants and support staff can check an individual's background, including convictions for crimes, especially sexual ones, and can weed out potential abusers if they attempt to get work within agencies that support vulnerable individuals. Megan's Law (1994), which requires known sex offenders to register, can raise awareness in a community. This type of law exists in all states now, but the registration was the result of a molestation and murder of a 7-year-old named Megan Kanka in New Jersey.

TOWARD MATURE RELATIONSHIPS

As people with intellectual disabilities mature toward full adulthood, the gap between biological maturity and social, educational, and emotional maturity seems to narrow somewhat. Thoughts about adult lifestyles and activities are brought into focus through transition planning and post–high school educational programs and vocational experiences. The experiences that have been available in friendships can be the building blocks for more adult relationships that might include romance and sexual intimacy. Social negotiation with friends about where to go to eat, whose turn it is in a board game, how to express personal interests and desires, and how to take responsibility for the maintenance of a mutual relationship become increasingly important as skills to apply to more independent, intimate relationships.

This is not to say that everyone with an intellectual disability can manage or wants an adult romantic relationship in which marriage, sexual intercourse, and perhaps a family are goals for the couple. Sometimes just being someone's sweetheart is most important. Sometimes having a date for the prom or a partner to dance with is what romance is all about. Sometimes a mutual sexual partnership is enough of a relationship to be satisfying. Sometimes a person wants and can manage being the sweetheart of another person while continuing to live either with their nuclear family or in a group living arrangement. Other times a person might be more interested in being a bride or a groom and having an elaborate wedding reception than in the marriage responsibilities and sexual options that are implied in that ceremony. Each individual and his or her family needs to realistically assess and plan for a future that will be satisfying, of high quality, and formed from the wishes, capacities, and values of the individuals involved.

If an adult with intellectual disabilities is perceived and treated as a child despite being a mature adult, it can be a lengthy and perhaps painful process for family members to change their vision. For families with typically developing children, the process of helping their children move from childhood dependence to marriage or adult relationships can take 20 or 30 years. Because there is a developmental delay for children with intellectual disabilities, their families often experience a developmental delay, too. It may take longer for families to recognize their child as a full adult with adult sexual drives and goals. Families of children with intellectual disabilities are likely to know much more about their children's personal issues and errors than families of typically developing children of a similar age. They generally want and need to be more protective of their children for a much longer time span. Parents recognize the damage that can be done by taking steps toward independence too quickly and know from experience that it will be their job to undo or mitigate any difficulty that their adult child causes or is the object of, especially sexual abuse or an unwanted and unplanned pregnancy. Sometimes family members become codependent with their children and have difficulty separating from their tightly bonded relationship.

Parents of adults with intellectual disabilities often are fearful that their child's interest in a mature relationship with a person of the opposite sex will lead to pregnancy and a baby that these aging parents will be forced to raise or that the added responsibility of a child into the marriage relationship will place onerous responsibilities and distress upon a fragile couple. While there is reality to that fear, it is not usually insurmountable. Some families welcome the addition of a new generation and are delighted at the prospect of grandparenthood and joyfully anticipate great involvement in the life of this new family member. Other times community social agencies, religious organizations, and service groups are willing and able to provide supports for a couple that has no family involvement or resources of its own.

But most of the time, usually with counseling and education, couples dealing with intellectual disabilities recognize how difficult it is just to take care of each other and choose to reject parenthood. They discover that the "Hollywood" version of parenthood is not reality. They learn that babies throw up, cost a great deal, limit other social opportunities, and grow up to be teenagers. They learn that children become more difficult to manage as they grow up. They learn that failure to provide for their child will cause them to lose their child for abuse or neglect or endangerment of a minor. Birth control that is situation appropriate, temporary, or permanent, is usually available and offers a solution to the risk of an unwanted pregnancy.

In today's world, not everyone gets married, has 2.3 children, and lives in a home with a picket fence. There are more lifestyle choices that are considered mainstream and acceptable even in conservative communities. Because we know that learning, growth, and maturity continue throughout a life time—and that our lifetimes are getting longer because of nutrition, medical care, and awareness of destructive factors in life—just because a person may not be able to manage sexual independence at a typical age does not mean that this is not a future goal that can become desirable and achievable with time and support.

CONCLUSION

Although sexuality begins before birth, we really begin to pay closer attention to formal sexuality education as children mature and are held less close to the family. Because children are beginning puberty at younger ages than ever, the disparity between chronological age maturity and maturity in other areas is even greater among youth with developmental or intellectual disabilities. This means that a person who may be physically mature and have typical age drives and emotions may not have the intellectual ability or social and emotional maturity or education and experiences to act in a way that a same-age peer would be expected to act. Consequently, youth and adults with intellectual disabilities usually require more guidance, support, and protection than same-age peers without disability.

A meaningful sexuality education that is tailored to reflect a person's specific learning characteristics and the necessary time and opportunity to accomplish these tasks is required. The range of social and sexual experiences for young people with an intellectual or developmental disability is likely to be significantly more limited than the experiences that a typically developing same-age peer has had. Youngsters and adults with intellectual disabilities are often dependent on parents and other trusted adults, such as pediatricians, teachers, older or more capable siblings, school counselors, scout or youth group leaders, or special recreation support staff, for guidance and support in making decisions involving sexual expression and avoiding high risk or potentially dangerous sexual situations. Trusted adults can help individuals with intellectual disabilities refrain from taking some of the unnecessary risks that are associated with adult sexual activity.

The importance of sexuality education for this group cannot be overemphasized for not only safety but also quality of life and a positive outlook for a full and satisfying adulthood.

REFERENCES

American Academy of Pediatrics Committee On Children with Disabilities. (1996). Sexuality education of children and adolescents with developmental disabilities. *Pediatrics, 97*(2), 275–278.

Baladerian, N. (Speaker). (2003). *Voices ignored* [CD]. Columbia: The Center for Child and Family Studies, University of South Carolina.

Being with People: Being with friends(1990). [Videotape]. Santa Barbara, CA: James Stanfield Company.

Brody, J. E. (1999, November 30). Yesterday's precocious puberty is norm today. *The New York Times*, p. F8.

Cohen, W.I., Nadel, L., & Madnick, M.E. (Eds). (2002). *Down syndrome: Visions for the 21st Century.* New York: Wiley-Liss, Inc.

Couwenhoven, T. (2001, March/April). Sexuality education: Building a foundation for healthy attitudes. *Disability Solutions, 4*, 1–13.

Eshilian, L., Falvey, M.A., Bove, C., Hibbard, M.J., Lailin, J., Miller, C., et al. (2000). Restructuring to create a high school community of learners. In R.A. Villa & J.S. Thousand (ed.), *Restructuring for caring and effective education: Piecing the puzzle together* (pp. 402–427). Baltimore: Paul H. Brookes Publishing Co.

Mattis, N.G. (1994). Teaching young children about sexuality and AIDS. *Brown University Child and Adolescent Behavior Newsletter, 10*, 7.

Megan's Law, N.J. Stat. Ann. § 2C: 7–19 (1994 & Supp. 2001).

Melby, T. (2001). Childhood sexuality: Norway leads the way in publicizing a sensitive subject. *Contemporary Sexuality, 35*(12), 1–5.

Planned Parenthood Federation of America & American Association of Sex Educators, Counselors, and Therapists. (2003). Masturbation: From myth to sexual health.*Contemporary Sexuality, 37*(3), i–v.

Schwier, K.M., & Hingsburger, D.H. (2000). *Sexuality: Your sons and daughters with intellectual disabilities.* Baltimore: Paul H. Brookes Publishing Co.

Sobsey, D. (1994). *Violence and abuse in the lives of people with disabilities.* Baltimore: Paul H. Brookes Publishing Co.

Staub, D. (1998). *Delicate threads: Friendships between children with and without special needs in inclusive settings.* Bethesda, MD: Woodbine House.

Vandenbergh, John G. (2003). Prenatal hormone exposure and sexual variation. *American Scientist, 91,* 218–225.

Vander Zanden, J.W. (2000). *Human development* (7e). Boston: McGraw-Hill.

World Health Organization (WHO). (1975). *Education and treatment in Human Sexuality: The Training of Health Professionals.* Report of a WHO Meeting (WHO Technical Report Series No. 572). Geneva World Health Organization.

Young Adult Institute (Producer). (1993). *Friendship* [Videotape]. New York: YAI.

2

Six Key Components of a Meaningful, Comprehensive Sexuality Education

Leslie Walker-Hirsch

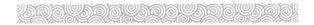

WHY DO PEOPLE WITH INTELLECTUAL DISABILITIES NEED SEXUALITY EDUCATION?

During his tenure as Surgeon General of the United States, Dr. Satcher's publication *The Surgeon General's Call to Action to Promote Sexual Health and Responsible Sexual Behavior 2001* identified people with disabilities as an underserved group in the area of sexuality education services. Many schools have sexuality education programs for their "regular" education students, but fewer school programs extend that sexuality education fully to their students with special educational needs. Although many students with intellectual disabilities are included in programs to the extent that they can benefit from them, there are some instances, such as sexuality education, in which specialized programs may be of greater benefit to them. For example, many students with intellectual disabilities are included in health classes, so they are *present* in class for the information, but they often do not get *educated* because the content goes by too quickly and is directed toward a group of students whose needs at that time in their lives are somewhat different than the needs of students with intellectual disabilities. For nonincluded students, the sexuality education often focuses on naming body parts, the biology of human reproduction, and warnings about the dangers of abuse and disease, but lacks the opportunities for demonstrating full comprehension and behavioral strategies that provide assurances of safety and ongoing supports in adult life situations. Adults with intellectual disabilities may not have any additional access to sexuality education or information once they leave their school settings.

In the book *Socialization and Sexuality,* Kempton (1998) described some of the reasons why individuals with intellectual disabilities need sexuality education. For one, the disability itself makes it more difficult for these students to gain the information and knowledge they need to develop a healthy and positive attitude about their own sexuality. In addition, individuals with intellectual disabilities often do not know who, how, or when to ask questions concerning sexuality because they often have inadequate knowledge or confused communication and thinking. They may have low reading ability and may not have easy access to books on the subject that they can read without an adult's help. Their friends may not be any better informed than they are. They may have been criticized or even punished for talking about subjects related to sexuality. There may also be little opportunity for them to observe, model, and practice appropriate and "cool" social/sexual behaviors in a nonjudgmental environment. Because their critical thinking ability and judgment are often impaired, students with intellectual disabilities have difficulty separating fact from fiction and myth from reality. These factors can often lead to problem sexual behaviors that are the direct result of being uninformed or misinformed about sexuality (Kempton, 1998). For example, a student who admires a movie star may want to express that, but instead of saying something such as, "Boy oh boy, she is so sexy!" he might say "She is my wife." Or, if a student is attracted to another student, instead of making light conversation, she may instead make an inappropriate sexual remark and be referred to the school disciplinarian and have her parents called to school. There are actually "flirting coaches" now available to teach people with social learning disabilities how to flirt, rather than get accused of sexual harassment (see, e.g., Heskell, 2001). Life coaches frequently include flirting as an important skill to use in almost any social interaction. These principles can also be adapted to meet the needs of those with intellectual limitations.

Sexuality education is an important safeguard for people with intellectual disabilities to recognize, prevent, report, and avoid sexual exploitation. Some people with intellectual disabilities try to use sexuality as a dangerous and inappropriate way to gain acceptance or attention. Many students with intellectual disabilities are likely to be overly acquiescent (they try to please by saying "yes," no matter what they really want; Finlay & Lyons, 2002), compliant (because they are taught to be docile and polite), suggestible, and dependent upon others for meeting their basic needs.

> Not long ago, a story of a special education student in an affluent suburb brought national attention to such acquiescence, compliance, and suggestibility. A young female teenager with an intellectual disability was invited to attend a party of sorts with a number of her male teen schoolmates. She was anxious to be part of this popular group and regarded them as friends, although she did not actually participate in typical friendship activities with them. She was known to be overly compliant, a person who would do whatever she was asked to do. While at the party, she was sexually assaulted with a broomstick and a baseball bat and was asked to engage in other sexual acts with these young men. She agreed and participated. A court judged that the men had used her intellectual disability to gain unfair advantage of her in a sexual manner. Despite the nature of these acts, she still regarded the men as her friends and expressed her concern that they would not remain her friends after her testimony.

Students with intellectual disabilities can have poor social judgment and difficulty in predicting the consequences of their acts. They are often sought as victims, not because they dress in a provocative way or because they hang out in unsavory places, but because they are viewed as less reliable reporters of abuse and less likely to be believed because they may not be able to tell a cogent story (Ellis & Luckasson, 1985; Sobsey & Mansell, 1994).

The goals of a sexuality education program for individuals with intellectual disabilities are to

- Support social acceptance
- Achieve greater social competence
- Enhance quality of life
- Reduce the risk of sexual exploitation
- Prevent the transmission of sexually transmitted diseases

Sexuality education can help individuals with intellectual disabilities in many ways. First, it can help them talk without embarrassment about their sexual needs and can assist them to make better decisions about what sexual expressions are within their ability to access. Second, sexuality education can help individuals avoid sexual abuse, disease, and unwanted pregnancies. And third, sexuality education can help individuals clarify their own values and desires and take personal responsibility for their actions. The greater the degree of competence a person achieves, the more opportunities become available. These opportunities can lead to a richer life experience and higher life satisfaction.

WHAT COMPONENTS OF A SEXUALITY
EDUCATION PROGRAM WILL ACHIEVE THESE GOALS?

There are six key components in sexuality education that support the development of sexually healthy children, teens, and, eventually, responsible adults.

1. Adult self-care
2. Anatomy and physiology
3. Empowerment
4. Relationship skills
5. Social skills
6. Social/sexual rights and opportunities

Education limited only to some of these components can lead to misunderstandings and mistakes, and may make individuals with intellectual disabilities more vulnerable to criticism or to being taken advantage of, instead of helping them become more socially included and capable.

It is useful to think of each of these six components as individual spokes on a bicycle wheel. If all of the spokes are present and they are given a chance to work, the wheel rolls smoothly. If one or more spokes are missing, the wheel can still roll, but the ride will not be smooth or safe!

Jessica is in high school. Last semester, she took a typical course in sexuality education that placed a heavy emphasis on personal hygiene, naming body parts, fearing strangers, and accumulating significant amounts of factual information about anatomy. Jessica was sometimes too busy to effectively manage hygiene during her menstrual period; however, the sexuality education program drove home the importance of practicing good hygiene throughout the day as an important aspect of her education. And Jessica was a good learner.

One afternoon, Jessica was stuck at the local grocery store for several hours because of rainy weather and her desire to avoid getting wet on her walk back home. She remembered that she should change her pad when she had her period and how important that was, so she went to an aisle in the grocery store and proceeded to do just as she was taught: She changed her pad, much to the surprise of the store manager and the other customers. Jessica became quite embarrassed once she understood her error in judgment. The sexuality education class she had taken neglected to help her practice problem solving, nor did it teach her proper situational etiquette. Although she had much factual information, Jessica had not developed the skills to use that information effectively to become more competent and have greater acceptance in the community where she lived.

Some of these components are concrete, require a low level of adaptive behavior skills, and are no longer very controversial for people with disabilities to learn about. Others are very abstract, require ongoing adaptation of social behaviors, and remain controversial. Some people erroneously view these components as beyond the scope and ability of people with intellectual disabilities or persist in believing the myth that it is a good idea to keep people with disabilities ignorant about sexuality for their own protection.

KEY COMPONENT 1: ADULT PERSONAL CARE

The first component of meaningful sexuality education is a focus on independent adult personal self-care. Adult self-care refers to dressing, toileting, grooming, and sexual hygiene practices. This is a standard and concrete area of sexuality education. Behavioral psychology has given us great insights into how to accomplish these goals using task analysis, repetition, behavior shaping, and rewards for increasingly successful approximation and achievement of specific behaviors. Self-care is not a very controversial area. Most people agree that independence in this area is important and achievable for a large majority of people with intellectual disabilities (Hughes & Carter, 2000; Price, Wolensky, & Mulligan, 2002).

Although perfection in this area may elude some individuals, independence should be the goal for most. Sometimes it is helpful to alter a person's environment to support the achievement of independence.

Carolina is 23 years old and has a moderate degree of intellectual disability. She lives at home with her devoted father and his wife. After she aged out of her school program, Carolina attended a day program where she participated in a sexuality education program that included emphasis on independence in adult self-care. Shortly after this program began, she started arriving at the program site with red-rimmed eyes and had teary episodes throughout the day. Agency staff suspected possible abuse, and an investigation was launched, beginning with an interview with Carolina.

Carolina recounted incidents of her father scrubbing her genital area when she showered and her anger at him. She had learned that the other women in her class were not subjected to the eyes of an adult man and were not roughly scrubbed in the name of cleanliness. Carolina's father was questioned and admitted to this vigorous washing of his adult daughter because "she had to be clean down there." Carolina's care was his responsibility since her mother had died. He told of his need to make her socially acceptable and sanitary. He told of his fear that Carolina would burn herself with the hot water in the shower or slip on the floor of the bathroom when she got out of the shower. He said he was "doing the best he could." Carolina was disrespectful to him, threw her food at him, and cursed at him, and he had used mild corporal punishment in an attempt to control her behavior and as punishment for disrespecting him.

The agency reported its findings to the protection and advocacy unit. They found that this was not a case of sexual abuse, but inappropriate behavior in regard to a "family matter." The agency recommended educational interventions and were willing to fund them. The agency also checked the hot water temperature at Carolina's home, set it within the suggested anti-scald temperature, and assured her father that she would not be seriously injured by the hot water. The agency also engaged a visiting nurse to teach Carolina to adjust the water temperature independently. The nurse placed a mark on the wall with nail polish to indicate the setting that Carolina preferred. The nurse also checked on Carolina's ability to manage her menstrual care effectively and dispose of pads in an approved manner. The nurse asked Carolina's younger stepsister to help Carolina wash her hair twice a week at the sink until Carolina was able to do it herself. The agency psychologist was engaged to work with Carolina and her father to help them express their problems and emotions without using profanity or physicality. A staff person was engaged twice a month to provide respite care for Carolina while her father and stepmother had time to themselves knowing that Carolina was safe at home.

Everybody needs to learn how to take a shower and use the toilet in addition to related social skills, such as distinguishing the men's room from the women's room and remembering to wash hands after using the toilet. Using the appropriate alterations of the environment and selecting educational strategies that were right for both Carolina and her family were the means of achieving sexuality education and moving toward independence.

KEY COMPONENT 2: ANATOMY AND PHYSIOLOGY

The next component of meaningful sexuality education is a focus on sexual anatomy and physiology. This includes naming body parts such as penis, vulva, scrotum, vagina, anus, breasts, and learning the normal functions of those parts at a particular age. It is very important for individuals to know—and everyone is entitled to know—how their own bodies work, what parts they have, and how to name them. Sexual body parts are important body parts. These parts of the body are worthwhile, although we do not discuss them publicly most of the time. Medical anatomical terms (or even their slang equivalent) for sexual body parts may embarrass family members and cause them to avoid discussing sexual anatomy or explaining how these structures work. Family members may not even know the function of these body parts and may not want to reveal their own lack of sexuality education.

It is true that the words that refer to sexual anatomy are not words to toss around lightly, and people typically do not use these words very often. Individuals with intellectual disabilities need to be taught that people typically do not discuss this aspect of themselves publicly and should be suspicious if a person they do not know well wishes to discuss their sexual anatomy or functioning with them. However, it is very important for individuals with intellectual disabilities to know sexual terms or their adult slang equivalent in order to talk about their bodies, find out if they are healthy or not, and communicate if they experience any sexual encroachment, abuse, or health issues. Knowing how body parts normally function can assuage a great deal of worry for youngsters, adults, and seniors as well.

Jeffrey is 50 years old and has a mild intellectual disability. Following his most recent physical checkup, Jeffrey reported that he had been sexually abused by his doctor who had been treating him for many years. He reported that the doctor raped him by inserting his finger into Jeffrey's anus. Jeffrey had learned that was a way in which men can get raped.

After some discussion, it was ascertained that Jeffrey had recently turned 50, and at this age it was routine for the doctor to digitally examine his prostate gland. Jeffrey was reassured that this was a procedure to protect his health, but it certainly would have been easier if the doctor had informed Jeffrey of this additional aspect of medical protocol and sought his verbal permission before proceeding with the examination.

Fortunately for Jeffrey, he had the personal courage and information to know that he should report his belief that he was molested. Some worst-case scenarios might have been any of the following:

- Jeffrey might have struck the doctor to protect himself from a perceived assault and been arrested or labeled as a person with aggression issues.
- Jeffrey might have believed that he was a victim of sexual assault and spent the next years of his life acting as if he actually was a victim, perhaps requiring psychiatric or psychological treatment.
- Jeffrey might have just refused to ever go to a doctor again because of a loss of trust for that whole group.
- Jeffrey might have retold his story in a more indirect way by repeating the experience with other men he knew.

It is important to know that sexual parts have other functions besides reproduction. Biology teachers in high school teach about the respiratory system, the digestive system, and the reproductive system. For most people, reproduction is not the main purpose of their sexual system. Often, more important sexual goals include emotional intimacy, physical closeness, the personal enjoyment of one's own body or the enjoyment of pleasing another person, and recognizing and reporting sexual health concerns. These sexual functions, however, are not usually discussed by the science teacher or the special educator. Most likely, neither science teachers nor special education teachers have had training in sexuality education for their special education students and are at a loss for discussing these issues within the school curriculum guidelines.

Ironically, health education or family life education teachers who do have training in discussing such sensitive issues probably do not have training in working with students with intellectual or developmental disabilities and do not have experience or information about selecting specialized educational materials or methods of instruction (Watson, Griffiths, Richards, & Dykstra, 2002). Discussion of specific sexual pleasures may be off limits in school curricula, and there may be no further opportunities for students with intellectual or developmental disabilities to access sexuality education in their adult lives.

As puberty approaches, the need for information about growing up becomes acute! As noted in Chapter 1, there is evidence that puberty happens earlier than ever before, more than a year earlier than a generation ago on the average (Brody, 1999). As children approach puberty, typical maturity-related changes in anatomy and physiology will take place. Typically developing children talk to their friends or their older siblings or they read books, stories, and magazine articles about growing up. If a child is not well prepared in anticipation of these exciting changes, the changes can be frightening. Children with intellectual disabilities, however, are often not prepared.

Imagine a girl who knows little or nothing about menstruation. One day, blood comes from a place on her body that she cannot see and that may not even have a name! She may assume that she is injured or ill. Or, imagine a boy who has finally achieved hard-won success with toilet training and has a wet dream for the first time and does not understand what it is. He may be worried or ashamed that he has regressed in his toileting accomplishment, or he may be fearful of disappointing his family when they discover his wet underwear or pajamas.

Youngsters with intellectual disabilities typically experience puberty around the same time as their typically developing peers; however, children with intellectual disabilities are likely to be delayed in the social and emotional maturity that typically accompanies this new stage of growth. This dissonance between biological maturity and social/emotional maturity often requires additional attention.

Many schools have begun educating students with intellectual disabilities about sexual anatomy in preparation for some of the physical changes of puberty. For example, teachers may discuss a boy's anticipation of shaving like his father or using deodorant regularly, in addition to the fact that he will begin to notice hair growth on his body. Teachers may show girls menstrual hygiene products and discuss their use, in addition to telling them about getting a more adult figure because their breasts will grow or even using models to describe the internal workings of female organs that produce a menstrual cycle. Even though this information is oftentimes shared by teachers, it is still important for parents and family members to corroborate this information, to reassure their child, and to support the behavior training hygiene that is involved in menstrual care and after wet dreams or ejaculation. It is also important to allow children to enjoy or be annoyed by these events and provide them guidelines related to these very adult experiences.

Juarez is now a 15-year-old teen with cerebral palsy and a mild intellectual disability. When he was 8, he began learning about the changes of puberty in his school health program. He learned that boys will eventually get hair on their faces and will need to decide about growing a beard or a mustache or shaving the hair off. Juarez and other students were reassured that their fathers were once boys who did not have facial hair or need to shave. Juarez said he was not going to have hair on his face and would not ever need to shave and that no one would be able to make him. The teacher did not press the point but moved along with the lesson. Recently, the teacher received a letter from Juarez's parents with a picture of him with white lather all over his face, shaving independently!

Public expectations of people change when adolescents present themselves as adults. The latitude that is extended to children who exhibit bad manners or privacy errors about their person or their spoken language is denied to adults for whom greater social skills are expected. The same holds true for young adults with disabilities. Inappropriate social and sexual behaviors or disclosures are typically readily forgiven when a child is the actor; but, ridicule, anger, and revulsion are likely community reactions when an adult makes these errors. As teens with disabilities appear more adult-like, more is expected of them by the people in the community in which they live, work, and play, and less digression is tolerated. Although the public generally holds a somewhat wider margin of error for individuals with disabilities, the accompanying pitying attitude can be even more difficult to bear.

The physical enjoyment of masturbation for teenagers and adults of both sexes is not something that is discussed in many schools. When Dr. Jocelyn Elders was the Surgeon General of the United States, she was criticized for talking about the "M" word, and some believe that she resigned her position as a result of this criticism. Most sex experts believe that masturbation, when done in private and for an amount of time that does not interfere with other important social and intellectual activities of life, is a normal, harmless, and ordinary sexual outlet. Sex educator Sol Gordon has said many times that if you don't like it, don't do it.

For many people with intellectual and developmental disabilities, masturbation is the only genital sexual outlet that is available to them. Each family needs to decide what guidelines are appropriate for them regarding masturbation and how to support both their child's desires and needs and the family's values. Parents can communicate values and preferences about masturbation and can insist on appropriate behavior in public, but whether their child follows that value when in private is up to the child and may not even be known by the parents. When there is conflict between individuals with intellectual disabilities and their families about masturbation in private, guilt, shame, and frustration may be the result for the child, and increased household tension may be the result for the family. Sometimes, an individual with intellectual disabilities will find other places for masturbation if he or she is prevented from having private time at home for this activity. The individual may choose to masturbate in the bathroom or in a stairwell at school, between two parked cars, or even behind a dumpster if he or she feels these are places where masturbation will not be discovered easily. These inappropriate and sometimes dangerous choices, however, are likely to cause problems when discovered or reported.

Youngsters with intellectual disabilities need to discriminate between private and public places. A trip around the house can be one easy way to specify those areas at home where privacy can be expected: either the bedroom or a bathroom with doors closed and windows covered. Having the opportunity to show other family members the private areas can help reinforce this important lesson. Although some degree of privacy can be accessed outside of the home for toileting, changing clothes, or medical examinations, there are no areas outside of the specified home areas where masturbation is acceptable. To help an individual with intellectual disabilities learn to distinguish private from public areas, parents can assemble a book of magazine photos and play a game of differentiating private from public areas by placing a purple dot sticker on the photos of private locations and to set the stage for associating a purple circle with privacy. This is a readiness activity for the CIRCLES®[1] curriculum that will further define social/sexual discrimination skills (Walker-Hirsch & Champagne, 1993, 2005).

---

[1]The registered trademark CIRCLES® and the descriptive materials herein drawn from copyrighted material in The CIRCLES® Series are used with the expressed permission of James Stanfield Company. All rights reserved. Duplication in any form is prohibited. For information about the CIRCLES® Video Series, contact James Stanfield Publishing Company, 800-421-6534 or visit www.stanfield.com.

Parents must teach their children with intellectual disabilities that it is not acceptable to display physically mature bodies in public and that the behaviors that relate to personal body parts must be performed only in private. It is important for parents to institute routines of privacy for the child and for other family members long before puberty is an issue. It will take some time to make the changes from childhood exuberance to modesty that is more adult, so it is best to allow ample time and not wait until the last minute to make these necessary changes. Anatomy and physiology, especially around the time of puberty, is an important aspect of sexuality, and sexuality education can alleviate some of the difficulties of puberty for children and their parents.

KEY COMPONENT 3: EMPOWERMENT

The third area of meaningful sexuality education focuses on empowerment. Empowerment is comprised of self-esteem, autonomy, personal preferences, values, and decision making. It is the force and confidence that helps us express our personal preferences and establish the direction for our lifestyle choices.

Empowerment is the ability to create the life that we want to have. People who have some control over their life choices are said to exhibit characteristics that are associated with good self-esteem, such as positive affect, polite social skills, eye contact, friendship skills, motivation, and others. Sharing decision making with a teen with an intellectual disability is an important step into adulthood (Hughes & Carter, 2000). It is important, therefore, for parents to begin to negotiate decisions with their teens and teach compromise. Parents must also help their children to see what choices and alternatives are available and what is likely to happen as a result of each choice.

Empowering people with intellectual disabilities has moved from a nonexistent practice to a controversial idea that has become less controversial in recent years. It is clear that it is easier in the short term to simply demand individuals with intellectual disabilities comply with the wishes and convenience of authority figures and yield decision making to others so that they can determine personal preferences for the individuals with intellectual disabilities. But this short-term convenience, however, is a poor choice for the long run. Assertiveness in expressing values and life choices is more likely to create a life style that is truly reflective of an individual's personal values and satisfactions.

Young people need to understand that what they do today has a consequence tomorrow; it can be a wonderful consequence or something they do not like. Opportunity to express preferences and practice in making small decisions with little risk is an important step toward maturity. First decisions should be about what to have for lunch or what TV shows to watch. These decisions should be respected and given support whenever it is reasonable. Criticism of these preferences should not be expressed unless there is likely to be a dangerous outcome. As the person with an intellectual disability matures and practices supported decision making with a trusted individual, he or she will gain more ability to make better decisions by understanding the consequences of the decisions. When more consequential life decisions are at hand, the process for making them will already be firmly established. This new competence to make supported decisions is likely to be a positive influence on the quality of those decisions.

Ramon is 15 years old and has a mild to moderate intellectual disability. In the past, he has been in some situations at school in which his vocational skills teacher complained that Ramon was not following the teacher's directions and that Ramon was being defiant by doing tasks his own way rather than learning suggested material. Ramon was referred for educational counseling.

During the education sessions, the teacher wanted to help Ramon express preferences and execute choices. Ramon and the teacher worked in a nonthreatening way, and the teacher asked Ramon to write down and draw his favorite flavor of ice cream, his favorite sport, and his best friends. He chose chocolate for ice cream, ice hockey for a sport, and James, Bob, and Henry as his best friends. Ramon was very proud of his drawing and asked to show it to his father, who had accompanied him to the session. Ramon's father looked at the papers and said "Ramon, these are all wrong! Your favorite ice cream is strawberry, your favorite sport is swimming, and your best friends are Mikey, Hernando, and Arlene."

Ramon burst into tears.

Ramon's father was not aware that whatever Ramon said were his preferences at that moment should be respected and supported. His son was expressing his personal power in a safe setting, and his father had been so judgmental that Ramon was intimidated to believe that his own preferences were wrong since they were not the same as his father's.

It is no wonder that Ramon found the vocational teacher's class a safer place to assert his individuality!

The slow process of taking responsibility for decisions begins early in life. Even if a person cannot envision all of the alternatives or their consequences, support can be offered without taking away the person's autonomy, as long as reasonable safety is maintained.

Too often, children with disabilities have their self-esteem assaulted. And the teasing is often related to their disability or their sexuality.

Gloria is 13 years old and has Down syndrome. After years of having loved school and charming all of her teachers, however, Gloria suddenly refused to go to school or speak to anyone ever again. She was referred to a social development counselor for help. As the counselor got to know Gloria, they began some puberty education using drawings as support for language and to stimulate discussion of different issues of maturity. Although Gloria did not speak at first, she listened attentively as the counselor provided information about some of the drawings.

When Gloria saw a drawing showing the many different shapes and sizes of women's breasts, she suddenly began to speak! She told the counselor that three girls in her gym class told her that because she was in the resource room and because one of her breasts was larger than the other she was not a girl. The mean girls told Gloria that since she was not a girl, she could not go into the girls' locker room or the girls' bathroom anymore. Gloria did not know what to do. These girls were supposed to be her friends and she believed what they told her. Gloria was afraid to go to school because she was fearful of having a toileting accident since she could not use the girls' bathroom any more. Gloria was also worried about changing for gym class, since the other girls also told her she could not use the girls' locker room any more. The only way she could think to solve these problems was to avoid school. She was so ashamed of not being a girl that she could not even tell her mother. So she stopped speaking altogether.

After spending some time talking about what it means to be a girl or a woman and what breasts are in all their different shapes and sizes, the counselor helped to reassure Gloria that she was a girl and that it was a good thing to be a girl. As evidenced, sexuality either can be a source of self-esteem or of fear and self-hatred.

KEY COMPONENT 4: RELATIONSHIP SKILLS

The fourth component of meaningful sexuality education focuses on developing and maintaining relationships. Finding, cultivating, and maintaining a wide array of good relationships could be perhaps the single most difficult of human tasks. These are also tasks that affect overall happiness. We cannot live without relationships. And we cannot live *well* without high-quality relationships. There is little joy without friends, family members, helpers, acquaintances, or schoolmates—all of these are different kinds of relationships. The most important elements of our happiness generate from our relationships with others. Children, teens, and adults with intellectual disabilities can usually enjoy the benefits of such relationships. Early friendships and relationships with family members are excellent practice for developing skills of assertiveness, turn taking, social negotiation, compromise, empathy, and caring; all of which are important in safely managing and enjoying more adult and more intimate relationships in adulthood. After all, if you cannot tell your brother that it is your turn at bat in backyard baseball, what is the likelihood of being able to refuse sexual advances that are inappropriate, unwanted, or even criminal?

Practicing assertiveness in a safe environment, such as in a supportive family home or nurturing classroom, can build these skills. Incorporating the language of acceptance and refusal as well as giving permission and respect to differ in opinion or preference can be helpful in paving the way to using assertive behaviors in more complex adult situations.

Friendships in younger years and close relationships with siblings and other family members set the stage for the development of adult friendships and romances. Many people with intellectual disabilities want to have intimate sexual relationships when they are adults. When adults with intellectual disabilities are able to access and reason about important sexual information, they will be able to meet the standards necessary to become consenting adults. That means that a person with an intellectual disability can participate in sexual relationships as a full citizen. Some adults with impairments in their intellectual ability marry and/or are partners in sexual relationships. The effort needed to enjoy this aspect of relationships can be considerable. Professional and family supports can combine with individuals' commitments to each other in a synergistic way to create happiness in ways that at other times might have been unachievable. As the poet James Whitcomb Riley has written, "The ripest peach is highest on the tree" (Riley, 1911, p. 15).

George is 42 years old and has Down syndrome and a moderate developmental disability; Linda is 46 years old with mild developmental disabilities and a concurrent mental illness. George has loved Linda since they were in high school. Both George and Linda live in apartments with same-sex roommates with the support of a residential agency. Friends, family, and staff view them as a couple, although they do not have intimate sexual relations. For the past two years, George has been asking the agency administrators to help him arrange for his wedding to Linda. Time after time, he was referred for sex education, then to premarriage counseling, then to life safety education, then to vocational training, and then finally to fire safety training, but no one ever helped him to plan the logistics of his wedding to Linda.

One day his mother's voice mail was flooded with messages accepting the invitation to George and Linda's wedding! In frustration, George had taken matters into his own hands! He had placed an ad on the radio station announcing his wedding. He had reserved the church party room, engaged the minister, and invited everyone in the town to attend his wedding to Linda.

Their families finally realized that George and Linda were serious about their marriage and began to do the real work of supporting this relationship.

That meant helping them to find an apartment together, helping them to manage their personal finances and state and federal entitlements, and assisting them in making a more limited guest list for the ceremony and party!

Linda and George are still married and living happily together with the support of their families and the agency that finally took them seriously.

Even if an individual cannot manage an all-encompassing relationship, such as a marriage, almost everyone enjoys choosing or being chosen as a boyfriend or girlfriend. Relationships that are mutual, not abusive, and within each person's ability to process and understand add great pleasure and excitement to life.

The most successful romantic couples are typically those that have partners who enjoy each other's company, have similar intellectual abilities and worldviews, share some common experiences, and have similar or overlapping lifestyles. The "even playing field" minimizes the likelihood that one partner will take advantage of the other sexually or that the partners will have grossly unequal power in the relationship.

It is important for children with intellectual disabilities to have friendships with both typically developing children and with other children who have disabilities. The nature of childhood friendships often changes at puberty, however. Sometimes the typically developing friend is no longer in the same school or class. Or, the friends may find that they no longer have very much in common. Or, the typically developing friend is less able to tolerate diversity in relationships. Or, the friendship becomes a helping friendship instead of the peer friendship it used to be. Often, typically developing individuals have more independence at an earlier chronological age than individuals with intellectual disabilities. This may mean that a teen with an intellectual impairment is not allowed by his or her parents to do the same activities that the typically developing friend is permitted to do. Teens, young adults, and even older adults may require a combination of inclusive community recreation and specialized disability oriented social events.

It is important, especially for parents, to value their children's friendships with both typically developing and disabled peers. This will help to avoid a situation in which a child with a disability learns prejudice against others with disabilities or places too great a value on friendship with nondisabled peers. When it is time for romance, individuals with intellectual disabilities are much more likely to find satisfying partners with intellectual abilities similar to their own. If disability prejudice has been instilled inadvertently, some excellent opportunities for happiness will not be readily available. Most of the time, being with a diverse network of people is advantageous, but it is also important to stay connected to others who have had similar experiences to your own and who share that culture.

This is not to say that every relationship that is romantic leads directly to sexual intercourse. Sometimes simply being chosen as a boyfriend or girlfriend and holding hands is a satisfying limit to sexual expression. Other times passionate hugging and deep kissing reflect the emotion of the relationship. Or even a chance to go to a family holiday event with a date fulfills a need to be recognized as an adult and as desirable by the opposite sex. These are opportunities that are not as available to many teens and adults with disabilities. And the opportunities that are available are not always sufficiently diverse or frequent enough to satisfy every need. Every state has different laws related to a person's ability to give consent to sexual interaction. These laws are frequently an attempt to balance a person's right to sexual expression with the person's need for protection from harm that may result from that activity. The American Association on Mental Retardation published a book called *A Guide to Consent*. The chapter concerning sexual consent represents state of the art minimal guidelines for achieving this balance. Since each state has different laws governing consent, there is no single document that clarifies the issue. However, all state laws agree that the need to have consent is basic to carrying out the aspects of a sexual relationship that are regulated by the law (Stavis & Walker-Hirsch, 1999). More details are addressed in Chapter 9.

Developing successful relationships can be a particularly difficult task for individuals with intellectual disabilities. Picture yourself with your friends. They all want to play Monopoly. You have never played before, but you are open to trying. You play a couple of rounds, but because you are new at this and do not know the rules or strategies, you lose every game. The other players are building hotels and houses and getting monopolies on properties, and you're going bankrupt every time. After a while you do not feel like playing anymore and your friends do not want to play with you either! It is no fun for anyone. How will you ever learn to play this game if no one will let you learn the rules or let you play without following the rules?

This is the kind of experience many teens with intellectual disabilities have when it comes to making and keeping friends and having and enjoying a boyfriend or girlfriend.

The CIRCLES® Curriculum Series (Walker-Hirsch and Champagne, 1992, 2005) is a widely used and successful technique to introduce youth and adults to the rules of the social world in a way that is fun to learn. The CIRCLES® curriculum is a multimedia program that uses many educational learning strategies to teach the abstract concepts of relationship expectations in a concrete and enjoyable way.

Walker-Hirsch and Champagne, the creators of CIRCLES®, theorized that they could apply some of the same proven successful teaching strategies to social development and relationship issues for people with intellectual disabilities that are used to teach many other aspects of academic and non-academic subject matter.

The curriculum uses videos, mini stories, visual support, discussion, paired associate learning, expressive art techniques, and role playing to convey the essence of a full range of relationship and positive and safe interactions. The life size role-play floor mat showing the CIRCLES® rainbow paradigm creates a safe practice environment for social interactions (see Figure 2.1).

The CIRCLES® schematic takes the abstraction of personal space and relationship boundaries and makes them concrete and specific. Each person is the center of all the circles, not unlike the sun and all the planets. The rainbow design is all around each person all the time, even if it cannot be seen. So, not only are you the most important person, so is everyone else. Everyone is important! The most important center circle embodies the self, self-esteem, autonomy, and empowerment; it is the place that is just for you. You are the most important person of your world of CIRCLES® and consequently you are the center of all the circles. The center circle is color-coded purple because that is the color for royalty. You deserve to be treated like a king or queen. An iconic sign is paired with the purple color and designates the Private Purple CIRCLE®. The message is that your body is your own and private. You decide who will come close and who will stay away. You decide who will touch you and who cannot. There is a domain of privacy each person has and can learn to access, as well as possessions that are important and private to that person. Thoughts, emotions, and experiences can be private, too. Each person has a part of himself or herself that others will never know.

Around that circle and touching it is another circle. It is not very big, but surrounds the Purple Private CIRCLE®. It is the Blue Hug CIRCLE®. It is the size of a hug. The iconic sign looks like a hug. There are just a few people who have this kind of closeness with us. For most people, the Blue Hug CIRCLE® is filled with loving family members. When we are adults, and if we are fortunate, a sweetheart might enter that circle and fill the sweetheart spot. A person should be able to name all of the people with that kind of closeness to him or her. While each of us has a blue hug circle and relationships, the actual individuals who fill that circle will be different for each of us.

Part of learning the CIRCLES® concept involves creating an individual set of circles that specifies who is actually filling that relationship circle in real life. The boundary of a blue hug relationship is illustrated in a high interest, low complexity video across the parameters of touch, talk, and trust.

Around that circle is another one, a little bit less intimate, a little further away, and inclusive of more people. Usually friends, extended family members, or people who act like family members populate this circle. This is the Green Far Away Hug CIRCLE®. Creating expectations for friends and extended family for touch, talk, and trust assists the person to recognize encroachment and potential abuse, perhaps at a time before harm can be done.

Sometimes, when it is time to fill in the names of friends, it becomes apparent that a person has no one to fill in. Although it is sad to hear that someone has no friends, it may be the first step toward discovering the obstacles to friendships and addressing them.

Around that circle is another circle, the Yellow Handshake CIRCLE®. It represents the social distance for acquaintances. A person whose name you know and who knows your name qualifies for that circle. We can shake hands but limit our touch to hands only. Similarly, there is more remote conversation, and less trust. There are usually many people in this circle. They are people you only know slightly.

Around that circle is another circle, the Orange Wave CIRCLE®. There is no body contact or touch in this more distant circle. You can see a familiar face across the street and just wave. It is best to wave to children you don't know well. It is up to their parents to decide who touches their children.

Around that there is the Red Stranger Space®. Most of the people in the world fit in this space. Most people are strangers; we do not touch them; we do not talk to them; we do not trust them. And they do not touch, talk, or trust us either. The exception in this group is the community helper. A community helper can be recognized by the badge or uniform that is worn, and by the specialized work-type setting. You can talk to the community helper about business. It is important to recognize what the limits are in business touch, business talk, and business trust for various community helpers.

The CIRCLES® program can be personalized according to the age and ability of the individual. The CIRCLES® guide book gives suggestions for activities that support the large array of concepts that can be addressed through the use of the CIRCLES® concept.

The two final components of a meaningful sexuality education for people with intellectual disabilities focus on social skills of sexuality and social and sexual rights and opportunities. These areas are still the most controversial and, probably for that reason, are still somewhat underdeveloped in many schools and agencies.

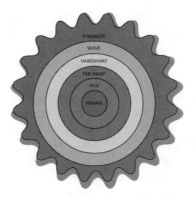

Figure 2.1 CIRCLES® rainbow paradigm.

KEY COMPONENT 5: SOCIAL SKILLS

Social skills are the behaviors and conventions that let others know what we want while we remain likeable. It is no trick to threaten another person and then get what you want from them, but it is socially unskilled and dislikeable. The person might get what he or she wants, but will be considered a social pariah and labeled *persona non grata!* And certainly not a person to trust as a friend or intimate partner.

Good social skills are passports to acceptance in community settings and they provide common *phatic* language (i.e., language that has little content in its words, but that communicates). For example, when a person says "Wow, today sure is hot!" what they are trying to communicate is "I am a nice person. Here is how my voice sounds. I know that I want to make contact with you and show that we are sharing an experience." Among people who do not know each other well, this verbal contact can be a beneficial social skill. Public social skills, such as saying "please" and "thank you," using a tissue to stop a runny nose, saying "hello" and "goodbye," and knowing how to set the table, are everyday social skills that parents and teachers want their children to learn. Most families teach these skills to their children directly by providing opportunities for children to model parents and older siblings. Typically developing children are able to screen out unimportant or extraneous material from a social situation and *voila!* they are replicating adult manners. Typically developing children often learn "schoolyard social skills" in a similar way. As if by magic they know which sneakers to wear, what backpack to carry, and what teenage greeting is hip at the moment. They watch their friends, high-profile classmates, or rock, hip-hop, and TV idols, and they copy their dress, language, manners, and sometimes even values. (See Chapter 3 for further information on learning vehicles.)

Copying the socially skilled behaviors of another person might seem an easy task. However, it can be a difficult one for individuals with intellectual disabilities because they cannot always differentiate between the desirable skills that are worthy of copying and the undesirable ones that others display. Public social skills can and should be taught directly to children with intellectual disabilities, often with repeated trials and frequently with hand-over-hand instruction. Performing these skills independently requires that the learner be able to screen out unimportant aspects of the environment and select only the most significant segment of the behavior, ignoring the rest, and then selecting and enacting the right practiced response. It is usually not the best strategy to depend on the person with the intellectual disability to analyze a new situation on the spot and then figure out the best, or most appropriate, response using adaptive behavior skills. Indeed, difficulty in adaptive behavior skills characterizes the disability itself.

Parents and teachers can help to make this social learning process easier by teaching social skills directly and providing safe, nonjudgmental environments for refining and shaping the skills through practice and rehearsal. Highlighting the significant aspects of a social interaction for attention can go a long way in isolating the skill that is to be modeled.

A "buddy system" in schools can pair a typically developing student with a student with a disability. The "buddy" can walk that student through some of the "cool" manners that are popular at the time, such as when it is acceptable to use the school cheer, which rock star or group is "in" at that school and how to show that you know the songs, or when to wear a mini dress versus a tee shirt and tight jeans. Buddy mentors can help students with intellectual disabilities avoid social pitfalls along the way. Student "gatekeepers" (Condelucci, 2003) can escort special education students into school clubs or sponsored events and offer that student an inside chance to observe and practice teen social skills in an inclusive setting. Specialized recreation can create events where targeted social skills can be attempted with less risk of criticism. Older siblings also can be of great assistance in opening doors to included activities and guiding their sibling with a disability through the social demands of new situations.

These strategies work well for public social skills, but what about the more intimate social interactions that are conducted in private? What are the social skills associated with sexual expression? How can a person learn to select and flirt with a romantic attraction? How do you tell someone that you are interested in hugging that person? How do you communicate that you do not want to be kissed? Or that you do! Or that you do, but not right now . . . or right here . . . Or that you do not know how to "french kiss"? What do you do at a party? How do you go on a date? What are the skills of intimacy and lovemaking? How do you know if the other person wants the degree of intimacy that you want? What do you do if someone touches you sexually and you do not want that to happen again? How do you stay safe from HIV/AIDS? How do you know if you are in love?

These are difficult questions! When it comes to learning these and other adult social and sexual social skills, there are no opportunities to copy the modeled behavior of parents, teachers, or siblings. These intimate social skills are performed when no one is there to watch!

Curricula for special education/sexuality education can be used to teach some of these intimate social skills, but schools often have prohibitions about the subject matter and the degree of explicitness that is permitted in abstinence-only education programs. Teachers are reluctant and not trained to discuss the social skills of intimate sexual behavior. Personal values of teachers, families, and students may vary greatly about which acts are acceptable and which are taboo. Some parents have felt a keen responsibility to teach sexual intimacy skills and manners to their children when they become adults. Frequently, however, these skills are left to agencies that provide adult services if they employ a sexuality educator or another professional who wishes to undertake this responsibility. Often, the messages "Say 'no'" or "Never touch a person there!'" are substituted for developing better and more subtle social intimacy skills.

Television shows and movies often show inappropriate, silly, or dangerous social skills related to romance and sexuality. Children and teens with learning difficulties need help from parents or older siblings to decipher and process which parts of a program are unrealistic or funny and which are illegal and dangerous. Sometimes, teenagers with and without disabilities use sexual terms that they do not understand. A parent must create the opportunity for providing new information and be an "askable" person. This can help a person with a disability avoid many sexual misunderstandings and behavior errors. A parent who clarifies and explains a misused sexual term to his or her child in a way that is useful and that reflects the child's age, intellect, and social maturity can turn a potential reprimand into an enjoyable teachable moment. This should be the goal.

Inclusive settings offer students with intellectual disabilities a great array of exciting social interactions. This means that crushes, dances, parties, school sporting events, riding the public bus, and going out for fast food are now part of daily life for children, teens, and adults with intellectual disabilities. Direct instruction about both public and private social/sexual skills is crucial to the safety and well-being of individuals of all ages with intellectual disabilities. Parents, counselors, and teachers should create a safe, welcoming environment to discuss and develop the social skills pertaining to sexuality that are useful at each specific age, including adulthood. Specifics about teaching strategies will be addressed in greater detail in Chapter 3. Ideas for parents will be discussed more fully in Chapter 4.

KEY COMPONENT 6: SOCIAL/SEXUAL RIGHTS AND OPPORTUNITIES

And last, but not least, the final key component focuses on social and sexual rights and opportunities. What kind and what quantity of social opportunities are available, both inclusive and specialized, for individuals with intellectual disabilities? How much sexual opportunity and independence is appropriate to balance the right to personal freedom and the right to be protected from harm? What are your values? How do you balance the relationship scale between risk taking and personal safety? Or should you tip it? What are the laws in your state that apply to a person's ability to give consent to participate in sexual activity with another person?

These are just some of the questions that must be asked when considering social and sexual rights and opportunities. Many still are unanswered at the moment. And perhaps there is no single answer to any of these questions! So much depends on the values of the individual and the person's commitment to learn what is needed to be safe as well as happy in their personal expression of sexuality. The ability to consent to sexual contact and the role of the law as it relates to sexuality and individuals with intellectual disabilities is discussed more fully in Chapter 9. Cultural differences regarding sexual expression are addressed more fully in Chapter 7.

CONCLUSION

The ways that the laws of our states regard children and adults with intellectual disabilities and their opportunities for sexual activity and expression will be discussed in detail in Chapter 9. However the right to a free and appropriate education to all children with disabilities has been guaranteed for more than a quarter of a century under the landmark law, the Education for All Handicapped Children Act of 1975 (PL 94-142), currently enacted as Individuals with Disabilities Education Improvement Act of 2004 (PL 108-446) (New Hampshire Education Law LLC, 2005). In today's world, sexuality education must be included under that aegis for the well-being and protection of individuals with intellectual disabilities.

The opportunity for individuals with intellectual disabilities to learn about sexuality, to date, to explore their sexual preferences and interests in safe and responsible ways, and even to marry are realistic goals for many people with intellectual disabilities. Goals are best accomplished with supportive parents, schools, and agencies in a climate of teamwork and open discussion. Without parental support for romance and appropriate sexual development, there is often a needlessly sad ending to many a relationship.

As mentioned previously, this is not to say that every relationship that is romantic leads directly to sexual intercourse. Sometimes simply being chosen as a boyfriend or girlfriend and holding hands is a satisfying limit to sexual expression. Other times, passionate hugging and deep kissing reflect the emotion of the relationship. Or, even a chance to go to a family holiday event with a chosen partner fulfills a need to be recognized as an adult and as a desirable companion. These opportunities are not always available to individuals with intellectual disabilities. Whether it is because transportation and arrangements are so difficult to make or because parents are reluctant to take responsibility for their own child and someone else's as well, failure by parents to acknowledge this aspect of life as normal, expected, and positive can hinder the relationships of individuals with intellectual disabilities. And the opportunities that are available are not always sufficiently diverse or frequent enough to satisfy every need.

As with typically developing peers, educating people with intellectual and developmental disabilities about sexuality can be difficult. It is important to always keep the lines of communication open and to understand that mistakes in judgment may be made. However, if a person with an intellectual disability is fully educated, perhaps some of those mistakes can be prevented or the number and seriousness of them can be reduced.

Do not forget to recognize how relationships enhance the quality of life for people with and without intellectual disabilities throughout life. At the same time, remember that a meaningful and comprehensive ongoing sexuality education is a necessity for enjoyment and safety in relationships and an important protection from abuse in relationships.

REFERENCES

Brody, J. (1999, November 30). Yesterday's precocious puberty is norm today. *The New York Times*, p. F8.

Condelucci, A. (2003). *Widening the circle of community*. Lecture. Retrieved September 3, 2005, from http://www.bianh.org/winter 2003

Education for All Handicapped Children Act of 1975, PL 94-142, 20 U.S.C. §§ 1400 *et seq.*

Ellis, J.W., & Luckasson, R.A. (1985). Mentally retarded criminal defendants. *The George Washington Law Review, 53*(3–4), 414–493.

Finlay, W.M.L., & Lyons, E. (2002). Acquiescence in interviews with people who have mental retardation. *Mental Retardation, 40*(1), 14–29.

Heskell, P. (2001). *Flirt coach*. London: HarperCollins.

Hughes, C., & Carter, E.W. (2000). *The transition handbook*. Baltimore: Paul H. Brookes Publishing Co.

Individuals with Disabilities Education Improvement Act of 2004, PL 108-446, 20 U.S.C. §§ 1400 *et seq.*

Kempton, W. (1998). *Socialization and sexuality: A comprehensive training guide for professionals helping people with disabilities that hinder learning*. Syracuse, NY: Program Development Association.

New Hampshire Education Law, LLC. (2005). IDEA Reauthorization. Retrieved May 19, 2006, from http://www.nhedlaw.com/idea%20reauth.html

Price, L.A., Wolensky, D., & Mulligan, R. (2002). Self-determination in action in the classroom. *Remedial and Special Education, 23*(2), 109–115.

Riley, J.W. (1911). *The lockerbie book* (pp.14–16). Whitefish, MT: Kessinger Publishing.

Sobsey, R., & Mansell, S. (1994). *Violence and abuse in the lives of people with disabilities*. Baltimore: Paul H. Brookes Publishing Co.

Stavis, P.F., & Walker-Hirsch, L. (1999). Consent to sexual activity. In R.J. Dinerstein, S.S. Herr, & J.L. O'Sullivan (Eds.), *A guide to consent* (pp. 57–67). Washington, DC: American Association on Mental Retardation.

The Surgeon General's call to action to promote sexual health and responsible sexual behavior.(2001, July 9). Rockville, MD: Office of the Surgeon General.

Walker-Hirsch, L., & Champagne, M.P. (1993). *Circles, revised 1993: Intimacy and relationships* [12 videos and multimedia]. Santa Barbara, CA: James Stanfield Publishing Company.

Walker-Hirsch, L., & Champagne, M.P. (2005). *Circles, Level 2: Intimacy and relationships* [12 videos and multimedia]. Santa Barbara, CA: James Stanfield Publishing Company.

Watson, S.L., Griffiths, D.M., Richards, D., & Dykstra, L. (2002). Sex education. In D.M. Griffiths, D. Richards, P. Federoff, & S.L. Watson (Eds.), *Ethical dilemmas: Sexuality and developmental disability*. Kingston, NY: NADD Press.

3

Foundations in Social Development Education and Sexuality Education Techniques

Leslie Walker-Hirsch

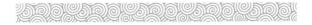

When I was learning to be a teacher in the late 1960s, I got the message that there was just one right way to teach a class: Anyone in my class who did not learn was considered a poor student. As researchers and teachers began to explore how children learn in light of the least restrictive educational alternative principle, it became clear to me that there were many right ways to teach, and that a good teacher had to figure out which was the right way to teach each individual student, regardless of how unique the student's learning style might be.

The advent of deinstitutionalization, community inclusion in school and adult life, legislation such as the Individuals with Disabilities Education Act (IDEA), and various special educational models (e.g., differentiated instruction, modified curricula, inclusive classrooms, individualized education programs [IEPs], developmental approaches to instruction) changed the definition of a "good" teacher forever. It became clear that students were going to learn the way that they were able to learn. It was now up to the teacher to figure out how to adjust his or her teaching techniques, classroom organization, and school environment in order to address students' unique learning styles.

Not only had teaching become effectively dependent on each child's unique learning channels, but it also became dependent on other variables, such as the child's age, the subject matter content, the child's specific learning strengths, the learning environment, both physical and affective, and the child's developmental stage of learning.

The term *developmental delay* has been used to describe several conditions that appear in children younger than 5 years of age whose milestones across a number of categories, including cognition, are delayed beyond the expected chronological age. A child older than 5 years of age or an adult with similar impairment is referred to as a person with a "developmental disability."

As an educator, I apply a developmental approach to special education as well as special sexuality education. As Greenspan (2005) noted in his research report for a comprehensive developmental approach to autistic spectrum disorders and other developmental and learning disorders, "Each child, even though he may share a common diagnosis with other children, tends to have his own unique pattern of development and functioning." To this end, a developmental approach should include "work with each child's and families' individual differences . . . in capacities to attend, relate, communicate and think and the capacities to process experience and information and plan and sequence actions" (Greenspan, 2005).

Accardo and Whitman defined *developmental approach* as

> The theory that people with mild mental retardation (cultural-familial retardation, retardation due to psychosocial disadvantage) without evidence of organic brain damage behave and learn in exactly the manner as mental-age-matched controls without mental retardation. . . . The developmental approach has been referred to as a motivational or social learning theory of mental retardation. (2005, p. 114)

As a special educator, I understand a developmental approach to learning refers to the way that a person gains information about the world and learns to function and behave in the world; a developmental approach to learning does not refer to a person's age; biological, social, emotional, or spiritual maturity; or capability. Such an approach pays less attention to the mastery of specific skills and more attention to an individual's strong channels for learning. A developmental approach should be applied not only to academic learning but also, and perhaps of greater importance, to social learning as applied to sexuality.

When a person's IQ is discussed, the person is sometimes categorized using the term *mental age* (e.g., "He is 25 years old, but has a mental age of 6"). The term *mental age* can be applied in a demeaning way, because it discounts so much that experience has to offer, but it is quite useful in discussing the developmental stages of learning and comparing the learning styles of students with intellectual disabilities to typically developing children according to Piaget's developmental stages of learning (Payne et al., 1981).

PIAGET'S DEVELOPMENTAL STAGES OF LEARNING

In order to individualize a learning approach for any particular student, regardless of the subject matter being taught, it is important to know some broad principles about learning and teaching.

A Swiss psychologist, Piaget, observed his own children as they grew up. He noticed that they approached learning situations differently at different ages. This observation led him to formulate a model of intellectual development in learning style, based upon milestones of achievement and linked to chronological age in typically developing children. (See Tables 3.1 and 3.2.)

Although Piaget watched the development of his own typically developing children in order to arrive at these classical theories, there are clear implications from a developmental perspective for effectively teaching individuals with intellectual disabilities. By assessing informally the developmental learning stage that a student evidences in his or her style and approach to everyday situations, a teacher can devise activities and lessons that will suit that individual's learning. These principles and learning characteristics apply not only to teaching academics but also to social and sexuality education for students with special educational needs. This same classical theory applies to teaching students the social development skills and sexuality education information and skills they will need to have to express their sexuality in safe, responsible, and satisfying ways within the law.

Once a teacher understands that a student will use his or her own developmental learning ability to gain information about the world, it becomes a challenge for the teacher to develop opportunities for that student to access information in a form that he or she is able to use. This understanding led to the development of the whole category of teaching called *special education*. Everyone can learn using special educational techniques, but some people cannot learn without them!

SUMMARY OF FREQUENTLY USED TEACHING STRATEGIES

There are many teaching and learning strategies that people use to transmit knowledge and information to one another. For those students with developmental or intellectual disabilities, some learning channels may be strong and some may be weak, blocked, or partially blocked. Special education teachers must create a specific educational strategy (e.g., lesson plans, supporting activities) to teach these students by appealing to that student's most effective learning channel or by strengthening a weaker learning channel with a specialized technique or device. The stu-

Table 3.1.   Piaget's developmental stages of learning applied to sexuality education

Stage	Mental age	Learning characteristics	Teaching examples as applied to sexuality education for those with intellectual disabilities
Sensorimotor	0–2 years	The person receives information about the world primarily through sensory and motor experiences.	Behavioral orientation uses basic reinforcers to encourage particular responses, to discourage others, and to shape prosocial behavior.
		The person responds primarily to intonation, rhythm, and context of language experience, not the abstract concepts that words represent.	Basis for teaching adult self-care skills such as toilet training, showering, and tooth brushing (Foxx & Azrin, 1973)
		The person is developmentally immature.	Uses menu of basic rewards, such as M&Ms, a cuddly toy, a whiff of a flower, a favorite musical tone or song, or a view of an attractive picture as reinforcers.
			Sexual self-stimulation (masturbation) is associated with pleasurable sensation but not erotic thoughts or fantasies (Planned Parenthood Federation of America & American Association of Sex Educators, Counselors, and Therapists, 2003).
Preoperational	2–7 years	The person begins to use symbols to represent objects and recognizes pictures as representing real-life objects.	Sexuality education relies on pictorial support for communicating information about sexual anatomy physiology.
			Teaching relies on concrete symbols and rules for specific behaviors, such as closing the door to the bathroom, labeling and expressing feelings, and discriminating private locations, private clothing, and private activities from public ones.
			Behavioral strategies such as task analysis are still important for learning support, especially when rehearsing new routines for modesty, using menstrual care equipment, expression of affection, anger management, sexual hygiene, and friendship skills.

Stage	Mental age	Learning characteristics	Teaching examples as applied to sexuality education for those with intellectual disabilities
Concrete Operations	7 to 11 years	The stage furthers the ability to order and classify objects and actions that are not abstract.	Teaching relies even more heavily on rehearsal and role play as vehicles for social learning, with extra practice on safe settings.
		The person categorizes objects and actions that can be seen or demonstrated.	The earlier strategies continue to strengthen understanding, especially in less concrete areas of sexuality education such as deciding what is right or wrong, assessing risks, evaluating the qualities of friendship, and the rules for dating.
			Social problem solving that is oriented toward independence is critical for this group. Using "social stories" expressed in verbal, written, and pictorial formats aids in self-efficacy.
			Opportunities for social and romantic relationships and mobility in the community begin to increase dramatically.
			Opportunities for "testing the rules" that exist among typically developing adolescents is an ongoing risk for this group until later in life when emotional maturity is more likely.
			Transition to the next stage can be a very high-risk time and can last for a longer period of time than expected.
Formal Thought	11 or 12 years and older	The stage encompasses the ability to deal with abstract, hypothetical reasoning processes.	The greater ability to use abstract reasoning skills within this stage create many more social and sexual opportunities.

(continued)

Table 3.1. *(continued)*

Stage	Mental age	Learning characteristics	Teaching examples as applied to sexuality education for those with intellectual disabilities
		The person develops the ability to predict consequences and to plan for various possible outcomes.	Complex social problem-solving techniques are needed because social and sexual situations may be more complicated and the associated risks may be greater.
		These skills continue to be refined throughout life.	Those with disabilities that affect social and sexual understanding may continue to need ongoing education, counseling, and/or support that is targeted toward specific situations that may develop.

dent's developmental learning level will then direct the choice of the activity. For example, if a child is trying to learn about sharing with a friend as a social skill, the teacher will have to decide how to communicate that concept. Can the child learn by actually experiencing sharing? Can the child listen to a story supported with pictures to understand sharing and transfer that knowledge into real life practice? Can the child read a story without visual support for black letters on a page and hypothesize how to plan for sharing tomorrow at recess? The teacher has to devise learning experiences that suit the learning of the child.

When the student's age and ability is combined with his or her most effective means of learning, *special education* takes place! And learning can be creative, easy, and fun for the student and for the teacher.

Memory

Memory is the ability to store and retrieve previously experienced sensations, perceptions, and information. Short-term memory is sometimes said to be a chronic area of deficit for a large number of people with intellectual disabilities, and it is thought to be a central factor in intellectual limitations. However, long-term memory is likely to be comparable among individuals with and without intellectual disabilities. Teachers are often challenged to help their students with intellectual disabilities move important information or skills into long-term, or even permanent, memory. Repetition is one way to help individuals with intellectual disabilities accomplish this (Ellis & Wooldridge, 1985),

Table 3.2. Summary of learning techniques

Name of learning strength	Definition of learning strength	Example(s) of using learning strength in social-sexual skill building
Memory	Ability to store and retrieve previously experienced information, perceptions, and sensations	Developing a sight vocabulary memory for signs and symbols indicating public bathrooms; using and remembering adult words to describe the experiences of puberty
Attention	Ability to orient to relevant stimuli and exclude irrelevant, competing stimuli in a specific environment	Using lighted visuals such as video to learn and practice selecting the essential elements of a social situation; actively engaging in social problem solving through role playing, artistic expression, or physical learning experiences
Motivation and positive behavior support	Ability to initiate and continue an action after the immediate stimuli is withdrawn	Having the opportunity to experience success at using a new social skill in a natural environment, such as the school cafeteria or gym class
Learning transfer: generalizing behavior	Transfer of learning is the influence of prior learning on performance in similar situations at future times	Learning to take turns when answering in class is generalized when the person chooses to take turns during a board game at home
Paired associate learning	Using information or skills that are already known to teach new information and skills by associating the new with the familiar	Using colored circles to represent social boundaries is a way to learn to discriminate different degrees of closeness in relationships (CIRCLES®)
Incidental learning and inclusive education	Absorbing information that is not specifically taught, but is present in a learning situation	Absorbing cultural traditions, recognizing the voice of a familiar person, developing personal mannerisms, interpreting facial expressions and using them
Imitation, scripting, rehearsal, and role playing	Learning by observing others and then practicing and repeating their behaviors and modeling their actions	Imitating the language of a parent, teacher, or pop culture icon can lead to social acceptance (or ridicule)
Positive behavior support	Using positive behavior modification techniques, such as tangible rewards, social praise, task analysis, shaping, and other strategies to reduce undesirable behaviors and maintain prosocial ones	A token economy that rewards appropriate classroom attire with privileges or objects of desire; offering increased independence at the mall can be used as a reward for compliance with appropriate in-store behavior

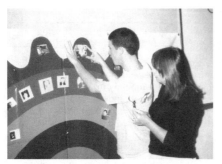

but repetition can become boring for both the teacher and the student. However, if the teacher varies the way that the same information is presented, students most likely will remain interested.

In social development and sexuality education for students with intellectual disabilities, the topic of sexuality becomes difficult for parents and teachers to ignore when children hit puberty. Puberty education can consist of a quick list of facts that describe the biological changes that happen to boys and girls as they mature. Every day, preteens could recite that list, be tested on that list, and be given a stamp of approval if they can recite that list after memorizing it.

However, if, in addition to a short list of facts, this information is repeated to students in various ways, they will more likely remember the experience of puberty education rather than just the list of facts, which is more likely to be forgotten. For example, in addition to memorizing a list of facts, it might be helpful for students to see a short film about puberty, look at drawings that depict both bodily changes and moods associated with puberty, see and handle menstrual care equipment, interview their parents about puberty and what it means to be more grown up, practice guessing the ages of people in magazines, create a poster about growing up, and/or use a journal to record their feelings. Successfully repeating the information can lead to continued interest and enjoyment, and better teaching and learning.

Emotional memories, such as those from intensely pleasurable (e.g., eating a particular dessert at a birthday party) or traumatic experiences (e.g., sexual abuse), are stored immediately as "flashbulb" memories and can last for a very long time. These memories can be to our benefit or detriment, but either way they are strong and enduring in long-term memory ("Posttraumatic Stress Disorder Sufferers," 2006). Intense experiences can create positive "flashbulb" memories.

Tom has severe intellectual disabilities. When I met Tom, he was 38 years old. The first few sessions we had together, he could never remember me, and he repeatedly acted fearful of my presence even though I had met him a dozen or more times. Tom would be soothed only after repeated reassurances of my kindness. We always ended our sessions with a neutral goodbye, but it was never a lasting reassurance for Tom. One day, we were paired up as a team to attend a Coney Point Amusement Park outing, and we went on a roller coaster together. After that experience, Tom still could not remember my name, but when he saw me, he said, "Coney Point! Coney Point!" and wanted to shake my hand. At this point, I knew that he remembered me! Our experience had made a positive and lasting impression in his mind, which included feeling safe with me.

Attention

Attention is the ability to focus on a specific target of learning while screening out all other environmental and internal distractions. Telling a student to pay attention has little value beyond the moment, if a student cannot pay attention. Special education suggests that highlighting the particular aspect of a situation that requires the student's attention helps to reduce the allure of competing stimuli and distractions.

Cuing a student about what to look for in a specific situation can help the student to focus attention on a desired target. For example, using pictorial, photographic, or lighted images (whether still or moving) can make attending to social development information more likely and can support learning for a student who is easily distracted. There is less competition for a student's attention when a high intensity image is presented from which to learn (Meador, Rumbaugh, Tribble, & Thompson, 1984). Seeing an image generally ensures that it is being processed, whereas hearing about a subject does not offer such great likelihood.

Gary is 32 years old. Recently, Gary attended a recreation day event with a group of individuals with intellectual disabilities, whose ages ranged from 12 to 35 years old. Gina, to whom Gary was attracted and who also was attracted to Gary, attended the all-day event as well. Gary and Gina spent time together at the meetings, at lunch, and then at the afternoon dance. When the dance ended, Gina's parents looked for her and found her in a corner of the dance floor kissing Gary passionately. They were shocked! Gina's parents sternly told Gary, "Seventeen-year-old girls like Gina are too young to be kissing like that with mature men like you, Gary!" The look on Gary's face made it clear that he had no idea how old Gina was! He clearly had not attended to that aspect of the relationship.

After the event was over, both Gary's and Gina's parents agreed that their children needed training to focus their attention on the age of any person who attracted them romantically.

Gary, for example, was cued to ask, "How old are you?" He learned that if a woman said she was younger than 18 years old, she was too young to be romantically involved with him. Using photos from magazines for practice, Gary also learned to estimate women's ages better. Focusing Gary's attention on age, building his skill in estimating age, and cuing Gary will likely avoid errors that could result in serious trouble.

Motivation and Positive Behavior Support

Motivation is the ability to self-direct or to continue self-directing when an initial motivation has been withdrawn. *Positive behavior support* is a motivating way to assist a person to reduce undesirable behavior and maintain prosocial behavior. A Functional Behavior Assessment analysis first determines what generates a particular undesirable behavior. According to the Oregon Department of Education Office of Special Education,

> Functional Behavior Assessment is a process of detailed analysis that seeks to identify problem behavior(s) a student exhibits within educational environments. Based on data collected through observations, interviews, and rating scales, it can give a clearer picture of the antecedents behavior consequences that may cause a behavior to be repeated. (n.d., p. 2)

The undesirable behavior is looked upon as a communication of a need in an unsuccessful way. Once the meaning of that behavior is determined, a behavior change or support plan can be developed that includes education and individual skill building, as well as altering the individual's environment, improving relationships, and monitoring health—all aspects of lifestyle quality. A reward menu is devised with positive tokens and/or privileges that are highly valued by the individual. These external rewards are earned for improved behavior (Association for Positive Behavior Support, 2006). The improved life quality is expected to make a permanent improvement in the positive behaviors of an individual after the frequent behavior monitoring and token external rewards are reduced or eliminated. Because the student has positive experiences resulting from more desirable behaviors, they are likely to want to continue to act in more pro social ways.

A person can be told many times that he or she is good at something or successful, but that is not as powerful as experiencing the feeling of success. Successful experiences help to develop the internal locus of control needed for ongoing behavioral change. Achievement of a desired outcome or accomplishment is much more motivating than simply being told "Good job!" While social praise can be motivating, it has been my experience that it is best used as an interim step until a specific short-term achievement can be attained.

Myra is 20 years old and has a communication disorder and a mild intellectual disability that affects her ability to sequence her spoken communications. She is very attractive and has repeatedly attempted to run off at the mall to flirt with male employees. After an unfortunate and inappropriate sexual encounter with a male employee, her family has refused to let her out of their sight and has curtailed her social activities. Now every day after school,

Myra has no scheduled activity, and she spends her time fighting with her brother and screaming at other family members, who also scream back at her. Myra screams until someone relents and allows her to do whatever it is she is screaming about, usually wanting to go out. The entire family becomes upset by these daily tantrums.

Myra's desire to have a more socially stimulating life and her family's desire for peace in their household worked harmoniously together to motivate all persons involved to support the reduction and eventual elimination of Myra's outbursts. Myra helped create a menu of desirable activities that she could earn by using adult communication to express her social needs. These were activities that could be carried out at or near her home and that would involve interaction between Myra and a family member, friend, or neighborhood adult. Making Jell-O, going to the grocery store, phoning a relative who lived far away, renting a video, working on an art project, and of course, going to the mall, were among Myra's rewards for adult social behavior.

Myra received stickers at scheduled periods throughout the day representing social behavior that was acceptable. If she received the maximum number of stickers for the required periods during the day, she got to participate in the desired social activity. If she did not use appropriate speech and resorted to a temper tantrum, her family members simply said they would not interact with her during the tantrum, and that she should talk to them when she could be more adult.

There was no punishment, no yelling, and no criticism, just motivation to achieve the attention of family members and the highly desired social activities that Myra herself had chosen as motivation. The temper tantrums stopped and social-sexual education about behavior in additional situations progressed using similar motivation. Trust was reestablished between Myra and her family as Myra took responsibility for her earning of that trust, which resulted in greater freedom for Myra. This became an ongoing cycle of motivation and success that was self-perpetuating.

Successful outcomes for positive behavior support relate directly to choosing individually valued rewards or motivators. It is important to recognize that what is motivating to one person may not be motivating to another! Reiss (2000) developed an assessment checklist that helps determine what is motivating to an individual and what is not by evaluating that person's unique preferences through the use of a scientifically developed scale.

Allan is 30 years old and lives in a community residence that provides 24-hour staff supervision with six other adults. At a recent annual meeting, all of the supporting clinicians and staff were discussing Allan's problems and had set up new goals for him. All of a sudden, loud snoring disturbed the meeting! Allan was sound asleep at the conference table. His case manager was upset and angry! He woke Allan and said, "What's the big idea? Here we are trying to formulate a positive program of support for you for next year and you are falling asleep, not even paying attention! What do you expect from this meeting anyway?"

Allan perked up and said, "This is the first time anyone ever asked me! Actually, I want an apartment of my own, I want to learn to play the piano keyboard, and I want a girlfriend to kiss and go on dates with!"

The whole meeting changed at this point. The case manager told Allan that there were a number of things that Allan needed to achieve in order to safely access that degree of independence. Allan said, "Name them and I will work on them instead of the stupid goals that you have described year after year that are not important to me!"

Allan's meeting was adjourned and a new date was set for a new set of goals that would be important to Allan. After more than one year of targeted and motivating skill-building tasks for Allan, ranging from cooking meals to showering regularly, he moved into his own apartment and began a band with himself as the piano player. He is still looking for a sweetheart by dating women he knows from work or from the dances at which his band plays. And, he is much happier and cooperative.

Learning Transfer: Generalizing Behavior

Learning transfer is the ability to use prior learning to guide actions in a new situation. Without the ability to generalize knowledge or skills from one setting to others that are similar at future times, we would always be starting from scratch. The ability to generalize behavior requires either social reasoning or the ability to learn rules and use them repeatedly. For a person with an intellectual disability who has rigid or concrete thinking, or with low achievement of social judgment, rote learning can at times be more effective than reasoning or applying abstract principles.

Certain situations can have such high risks that learning from trial and error or learning by successive approximations of behavior

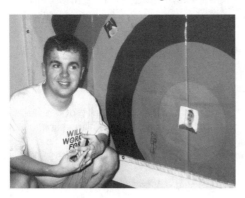

is too dangerous. In these situations, applying the same rules repeatedly without adaptation based upon judgment across all circumstances might be necessary to avoid great embarrassment or promote maximum safety.

The rules for sexual conduct often fall into these two categories: rote learning and social reasoning. What are the rules for changing a menstrual pad? What are the rules if a boyfriend or girlfriend hurts you? What are the rules about touching on a movie date? What are the rules for using a condom? It is useful to be able to always do the same thing, no matter where, no matter with whom, no matter what the situation.

There are, however, some serious pitfalls in relying too heavily upon rules to govern social and sexual behavior. Developmentally, a stage that occurs for typically developing adolescents has to do with testing the rules, to see if the rules apply as universally as they had been taught as children. As typically developing children move out of their teens and approach adulthood, their ability to use reasoning and to appreciate the subtlety of many social and moral issues increases dramatically. And the situations that they encounter as young adults often require this increased degree of judgment. For many individuals with intellectual and developmental disabilities, however, this growth in judgment occurs in much later years or to a significantly reduced degree. Young adults with intellectual disabilities are not likely to have the same social reasoning ability as their same age peers. Yet they may still be challenged to test the rules in order to participate in the same social activities and associated risks. In addition, the period known as adolescence, in which rule testing is frequent, is usually one that is prolonged among those with intellectual disabilities. Teens and young adults in their twenties often want to participate in social and sexual activities that their same-age peers do. Their intellectual disability and decreased development of social judgment, however, may subject them to risks that they may not be able to manage safely.

A frequently told urban legend among sexuality educators of youth and adults with intellectual disabilities is of a young man who was going out on a date and whose father wanted to be supportive of his adult sexuality. His father had educated him about condom use with an actual condom and a banana. The son reassured his father that he was well prepared in case a sexual situation developed since he had had done exactly as he had been taught. After the son left for the date, his father found a condom on a banana in the refrigerator!

Sometimes the wrong rule is called upon to meet the perceived demands of a given situation. For example, a few years ago, I was attending a self-advocates, conference on a very cold morning. I had arrived early and was not well known to most of the self-advocates. As one young woman came in from the cold, the static electricity of the dry air caused her dress to stick up to her waist. Wanting to help her avoid the embarrassment that would accompany this event, I whispered to the woman that her dress was caught up. She looked at me and replied, "I do not talk to strangers!"

When learning rules is essential, they can be coupled with other learning strategies to create an effective vehicle for mastery of simple social situations in a relatively short time. Be wary of using negative examples that show what *not* to do. This can create a circumstance in which the learner confuses what *not* to do with what is desirable to do. Extra practice, rehearsal, highlighting, repetition, social reward, and cuing can certainly reinforce a positive functional behavior routine that may allow access to a wide variety of social opportunities that otherwise might not be attainable.

Paired Associate Learning

Paired associate learning is the ability to associate known pairs—such as words and objects, names and places, and dates and events—to items that are new.

Mnemonic devices such as "lefty loosey, righty tighty" to remember which way to turn the screw top on the peanut butter jar, or the universal symbols for men's and women's public bathrooms, are examples of paired associate learning or pairing that many of us use. Singing the alphabet song associates a tune with the specific ordering of the letters of the alphabet.

Paired associate learning is the basis for color-coding objects or for many of those memory-enhancing courses for senior citizens with failing short-term memory. In special education, color-coding is an important nonverbal use of this pairing technique. The CIRCLES®[1] curriculum (Walker-Hirsch & Champagne, 1993, 2005), uses this pairing technique extensively to teach social boundaries. Each of the six colored circles becomes associated with a particular cluster of expectations in a relationship category. By associating specific colors with various relationships and further pairing them with expectations for touch, talk, and trust that is specific to each, navigating the complexity of the social fabric can become more manageable.

Incidental Learning and Inclusive Education

Incidental learning is the ability to learn what is not taught, but is also present in a learning situation, as if by osmosis. Although there are many high-minded principles that form the ethical basis for inclusion, there

---

[1]The registered trademark CIRCLES® and the descriptive materials herein drawn from copyrighted material in The CIRCLES® Series are used with the expressed permission of James Stanfield Company. All rights reserved. Duplication in any form is prohibited. For information about the CIRCLES® Video Series, contact James Stanfield Publishing Company, 800-421-6534, or visit www.stanfield.com.

are also educational benefits, especially in the social learning arena, for students with intellectual or developmental disabilities. Learning in an inclusive setting effectively improves social behavior because of higher expectations in the general education classroom than in the segregated setting, provides a rich support network, especially social support from classmates without disabilities, and helps teachers and students more flexibly adapt to learning and teaching differences (Kochhar, West, & Taymans, 2000).

An inclusive educational setting is a place where social behavior can be learned incidentally, by being present in the classroom and participating with others who already have greater social skills. Face and voice recognition, socialization style, manners, local slang, facial expression, and a sense of personal values are often learned incidentally at school. It is a person's whole environment that contributes to incidental learning. Exposure at school to bulletin boards, chatter in the play areas, classmates, and school and community events creates opportunity, knowledge, and skills that the special education student would have likely missed.

Television programs, movie stars, and sports and pop culture role models contribute to learning in an incidental way. Determining that it is "cool" to wear Derek Jeter's Yankee jersey because another boy at school had it on creates a common bond and an opportunity to identify with a group. What classroom items must be shared, how others respond to poor social behavior, how arguments are settled in the school play area, and how teachers praise or criticize a student's academic performance are incidental learning experiences, too.

A family home is another inclusive setting where incidental learning can take place. How affection is expressed by family members, the way that parents and siblings respond to sexuality on TV, and the way family members convey modesty are all absorbed as incidental learning.

Matt is 15 years old and has Down syndrome. Matt attends high school in a partially inclusive program where he learned the difference between appropriate school behavior and acting silly. He learned that he would be removed from the inclusive environment if he acted silly or inappropriate and would have to wait for the school principal in the office. This had happened several times, and Matt knew the drill. On a particular day, Matt did not want to attend speech therapy. He went into silly provocative dance gyrations on purpose. He had learned, incidentally, that he would be removed from the environment if he acted silly and would be required to wait in the office for the principal. He used this incidental learning to avoid speech therapy for the day. Inadvertently, his incidental learning ability had taught him a way to manipulate the teachers at school and spend his speech therapy period in a different environment.

When this was pointed out to the speech therapist, she adjusted her teaching. She asked that a "communication partnership" be formed between Matt and another student of the same grade. She incorporated speech and language activities into their conversations about subjects they had interest in.

In the social arena, the skills of friendship are often taught in an incidental manner to typical students and to students with intellectual disabilities, but friendship skills must often also be supplemented for those with intellectual disabilities with direct teaching that is oriented toward practice in a safe setting and scripting to develop an interactive routine that does not require frequent change or language planning, once it is mastered.

Matt continued speech and language therapy several times a week. He progressed nicely in his speech articulation, and his communication partner became his best friend at school. The friendship developed incidentally.

Teachable moments are more likely to develop in an inclusive setting that will be useful later in life in the postschool world.

Elvira is a 12 year old with a moderate intellectual disability. She was walking down the hall with the school librarian to become familiar with the route to the library from her homeroom. On the walk, Elvira noticed a gold bracelet on the hallway floor. She picked it up and began to put it into her pocket. The librarian used this unanticipated moment to discuss what Elvira should do if she found something of value that did not belong to her. They made a detour to the school lost and found and turned in the bracelet.

There are pitfalls in depending too heavily upon incidental learning. Sometimes students with intellectual disabilities do not know which elements in an environment are the most important and devote attention to stimuli and experiences that are of little value. An easily distractible student can have difficulty screening out stimuli that are not relevant, and learning can be impeded by incidental learning that supplants the learning that is intended.

Imitation, Scripting, Rehearsal, and Role Playing

Imitation is the ability to learn through the observation and replication of the behavior of others. It is also known as modeling or observational learning. Developing realistic role-play scenarios can be an enjoyable and creative way to compensate for a student who is slow to develop hypothetical thinking. The situations that a teacher or group leader might choose should reflect the student's age and complexity of thinking. Learning to call out "stop" as it applies to various situations can be practiced, with volume ranging from soft to loud yelling, depending upon the severity of the situation.

For students or adults who have difficulty with word finding, scripting to develop "tip of the tongue" phrases in response to a variety of likely social interactions can go a long way to increase social inclusion and friendly interactions. The student who has a number of scripted phrases can use recall to summon a good response rather than use reasoning to create new language each time a conversational opportunity arises.

Positive Behavior Support

Behavioral approaches to learning using positive behavioral strategies and supports reflects a person's ability to respond and demonstrate learning by modifying his or her behavior through the teacher's or therapist's manipulation of the consequences of the students' behavior and by creating an environment that supports the continuation of prosocial behavior.

Behavioral strategies and positive behavioral support are frequently effective techniques with those students with intellectual disabilities. Students with developmental delays, for example, often respond well to concrete rewards, tokens as symbols of accomplishment, and social approval. Many students with intellectual disabilities have greater external locus of control and respond positively to reinforcement that can be earned for performance or for meeting a set of well-understood expectations or goals.

Daniel is 13 years old and attends a segregated secondary school geared toward providing services to students whose behaviors are determined to be too difficult to be safely managed in a less restrictive environment. He has a mild intellectual disability, but that is not what is holding Daniel back in his progress toward inclusion. When Daniel has the opportunity, he befriends a female adult, usually a family member, teacher, or aide, and begins to ask at first innocent questions, then more personal ones, and eventually sexual ones that include requests that the female lift up her shirt or disrobe. Each time Daniel's sexual language began to escalate at home, his mother would distract him by giving him a small toy. So Daniel learned that if he wanted a new toy, all he had to do was begin sexual talk and he would be redirected with a new toy. When Daniel's mother did not give him a toy, he became physically aggressive. When he was a small child, physical aggression was not very hard to stop, but now that he was actually bigger than his mother, she was frightened of his uncontrollable aggressive behavior.

A behavior program was developed in which Daniel surrendered all of his cars and could earn them back through appropriate behavior. Daniel learned new conversation skills and was able to use more appropriate language to engage adult females. He received a toy when he had had a specified number of sex talk–free and aggression-free intervals. He was encouraged to expand his reward menu to include activities that he enjoyed and privileges that he desired as well. If Daniel was inappropriate he was given "the cold shoulder" for a short amount of time and could earn his way back to warmth by showing good behavior for a specified period of time. Daniel's inappropriate sexual talk was eliminated and he has made good progress toward managing his aggression as well.

Any and all of these learning vehicles, alone or in a variety of combinations and permutations, can be used successfully to teach individuals with cognitive disabilities at all ages and in a variety of settings. A teacher or a parent can be creative and individualize any learning task in a multiplicity of ways to arrive at a mechanism that will be effective for a particular student in a particular setting.

REFERENCES

Accardo, P.J., & Whitman, B.Y. (2005). *Dictionary of developmental disability terminology* (2nd ed.). Baltimore: Paul H. Brookes Publishing Co.

Association for Positive Behavior Support. (n.d.). *What is positive behavior support?* Retrieved February 4, 2006, from http://www.apbs.org/PBSTopics.htm

Ellis, N.R., & Wooldridge, P.W. (1985). Short-term memory for pictures and words by mentally retarded and nonretarded persons. *American Journal of Mental Deficiency, 89*(6), 622–626.

Foxx, R., & Azrin, N. (1973). *Toilet training the retarded: A rapid program for day and nighttime independent toileting.* Champaign, IL: Research Press.

Greenspan, S.I. (2005). *Research report for a comprehensive developmental approach to autistic spectrum disorders and other developmental and learning disorders: The developmental, individual difference relationship-based (DIR®) model.* Retrieved June 20, 2006, from http://www.icdl.com/selectedarticles/doc/ResearchonDIRandSEGC.doc

Hines, R.A. (2001). *Inclusion in middle schools.* Champaign, IL: ERIC Clearinghouse on Elementary and Early Childhood Education. (ERIC Document Reproduction Service No. ED459000)

Kochhar, C.A., West, L.L., & Taymans, J.M. (2000). *Successful inclusion: Practical strategies for a shared responsibility.* Upper Saddle River, NJ: Prentice-Hall.

Meador, D.M., Rumbaugh, D.M., Tribble, M., & Thompson, S. (1984). Facilitating visual discrimination learning of moderately and severely mentally retarded children through illumination of stimuli. *American Journal of Mental Deficiency, 89,* 313–316.

Oregon Department of Education, Office of Special Education (n.d.). *Functional behavioral assessment.* Retrieved June 2, 2006, from www.members.tripod.com/trainland/behavior.htm

Payne, J.S., Polloway, E.A., Smith, J.E., & Payne, R.E. (1981). Strategies for teaching the mentally retarded. New York, NY: Charles E. Merrill Publishing Company.

Planned Parenthood of Federation of America & American Association of Sexuality Educators, Counselors, and Therapists. (2003). Masturbation: From myth to sexual health. *Contemporary Sexuality, 37*(3).

Posttraumatic stress disorder sufferers store memories differently in brain. (2006). Retrieved June 20, 2006, from http://www.healthyplace.com/communities/anxiety/news/ptsd-memories.asp

Reiss, S. (2000). *Who am I? The 16 basic desires that motivate our action and define our personalities.* New York: Tarcher Putnam.

Walker-Hirsch, L., and Champagne, M. P. (1993). *Circles, revised 1993: Intimacy and relationships.* 12 videos and multimedia. Santa Barbara, CA: James Stanfield Publishing Company.

Walker-Hirsch, L., and Champagne, M.P. (2005). *Circles, level 2: Intimacy and relationships.* 12 videos and multimedia. Santa Barbara, CA: James Stanfield Publishing Company.

II

Sexuality and Intellectual Disability as a Cultural Phenomenon

4

A Parent's Perspective

Supporting Challenges and Strategies

Emily Perl Kingsley and Leslie Walker-Hirsch

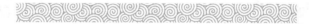

Jenny is 17 years old and has a moderate intellectual disability. Jenny's mother was amused when Jenny came home from her Friday night Special Recreation social group and announced that she had a boyfriend. Her mother thought it was sweet.

When a staff counselor called Jenny's mom and reported that Jenny and her boyfriend had been observed "making out" in the corner, her mother went into shock! "But Jenny is like a 6-year-old! She isn't interested in 'that sort of thing!'"

But Jenny WAS interested in "that sort of thing" and Jenny's mom had to rethink her approach to Jenny's social and sexual education.

INTRODUCTION

Not so long ago in approximately the mid 1970s, many parents and professionals, in a radically new approach, suggested that people identified as having intellectual and developmental disabilities could—and should—experience life to a much fuller extent than had ever been thought possible. They suggested closing institutions and encouraged a wide range of opportunities previously denied to these individuals.

The authors would like to give special thanks to Marklyn Champagne, Michael Goldstein, Cynthia Smalley, Christine Ricard, and the many parents who shared their thoughts with us.

These opportunities included being raised in their own family homes, attending "regular" local schools, working in their communities, becoming contributing members of society, and developing age-typical relationships. These new visions reflected true progress toward improved quality of care, individualized lifestyle choices, and expandedsocial/sexual opportunities. Broad changes to advance these goals are now legislated in many states.

This new attitude expanded opportunities in areas of education, community living, employment, and socialization. Along with advances, however, came new challenges that had not been dealt with in previous eras. Parents suddenly had to deal with their children's social and sexual development in the framework of a community environment rather than the sequestered setting of an institution.

Legislation was passed providing that students with intellectual or developmental disabilities should attend their local schools, attending as many regular classes as possible and only attending special classes to the extent needed. However, this legislation did *not* specifically provide for social education and inclusion as part of the regular school curriculum.

As a result, even to this day, it is often left to parents to provide these kinds of options, education, and experiences for their school-age and adult children with intellectual disabilities. Guiding a child through the turmoil of adolescence, social development, and sexuality education is a daunting task for all parents! Providing that guidance for a child with an intellectual disability presents additional challenges, which may seem overwhelming. Because these children and their parents have few precedents or role models to guide them or advise them, they may feel isolated, confused, and apprehensive.

Despite the difficulty of the task, parents have already committed to teach, love, support, and guide their children. Parents have experienced the pride and pleasure of each accomplishment and each step toward self-reliance and maturity that their children have achieved. They have taught them to tie their shoes, dress themselves, eat with a fork, and a myriad of other skills of self-sufficiency.

Parents and teachers often spend a great deal of energy and time on the academic development of children when they are young, while spending much less time envisioning what adult life will be like for those children. Concerns about adult life surface later.

As their children enter adolescence, it is important for parents of children with intellectual disabilities to remember that this is just another phase in their children's journey toward adulthood.The reality of a child's impending adult life pops into sharp focus when the physical and biological aspects of puberty appear. Parents often find themselves unprepared for this new set of challenges associated with new steps in maturity.

As with the other milestones and phases before puberty, parents need to take on this new topic with the same spirit of commitment as in previous areas of development. It will take work, but mothers and fathers will see the rewards of their efforts as their children gain confidence and become socially skilled.

TALKING ABOUT SEX CAN BE DIFFICULT FOR ALL PARENTS

In a personal communication on May 5, 2006, Dr. Iris J. Prager, Ph.D., past president of the American Association for Health Education, recounted that through her 20 years of professional experience, she has observed that a majority of parents—whether of children with or without intellectual disabilities—have a hard time discussing sexuality issues with their children. There are a number of reasons why this is so.

- Parents are often concerned that if they discuss sexuality with their children, it will imply tacit approval of adult sexual activities and even encourage sexual behavior for which the parent believes their children are not ready. The erroneous presumption is that if sexuality is not discussed, it may postpone sexual interest or behavior until a later date, when children may be more ready.

- Parents are often embarrassed to introduce the subject and language of sexuality into family conversations, especially at a time when their children are already sexually aware and interested. If a parent never had sexuality discussions with his or her child when the child was young, it can be uncomfortable to introduce the topic when the child is a teenager. Language for discussion, when it has not already been established during childhood, is more difficult to introduce when the child is more sexually aware and when silence has already been the established level of communication. The root of the embarrassment may also be related to the fear that the parents might be asked to share their own personal sexual experiences, activities, or preferences.

- Some parents find it hard to believe that their children are growing up and will be facing more adult decisions and having more independence before the parents are ready to relinquish their control.

- Many parents assume (or hope) that schools will take care of educating their children about sexuality. Parents may think that teachers have much more experience with teens and perhaps have access to better information and tools to use when discussing these delicate issues.

- Single parents who have children of the opposite sex can find it difficult to know what specific information their children need and when it might be needed.

- Parents may find themselves confused as adults in a world that is very different from the teenage world they remember. Mores, practices, and language, plus the increased visibility and pervasiveness of sexuality in modern culture, may make parents additionally uncomfortable.

- Parents are often not confident about the subject of sexuality. They themselves may not be sure that they have the correct information and terminology to provide sexuality education for their children. They may be concerned that they will give them misinformation or reveal their own ignorance. After all, most parents may not have gotten good sexuality education themselves from their own school or parents.

- Parents may also be unsure of just how much their children already know, whether correct or incorrect information. Children may even know more than their parents do. That is likely to leave parents even more insecure about their ability to guide their children in this important area of life.

- Parents may have their own personal issues that may interfere with communication or unintentionally influence the subtext and interpretation of the discussion.

In a recent *New York Times* article on puberty education, Dr. Stanley Snegroff, Director of the Adelphi University Graduate Program in Health Studies, observed, "It's amazing the extent to which communication between parents and children on this [issue] is still greatly lacking" (Bellafante, 2005).

IT IS EVEN MORE DIFFICULT FOR PARENTS OF CHILDREN WITH DISABILITIES TO ADDRESS ISSUES OF SEXUALITY

It is certainly clear that the subject of sexuality is a hard one for all parents. For parents who have children with intellectual disabilities, there are many other emotional as well as objective reasons for this difficulty. Addressing their children's sexuality is much more challenging and complex for these parents. In addition to issues raised previously, parents of children and adults with intellectual disabilities also have other overlays that often remain unspoken or camouflaged by reticence or fear. For example:

It is Painful to Be Reminded—Once Again—that Your Child Has Significant and Permanent Limitations

It is daunting for many parents of children with intellectual disabilities to continually confront new challenges with the knowledge that everything takes longer; requires more time, energy, and repetition; and is not guaranteed to succeed. Once a child has reached a certain level of accomplishment, some parents may feel a great temptation to stop or "slide" at that level, rather than undertaking new challenges and advancing their children beyond their current level of achievement. Some parents find it comforting to embrace the notion of their children reaching a plateau. Others resent that idea and see each level as a starting point to new challenges in the child's continued development. As a child grows up, the kinds of challenges he or she faces become more complex and complicated and have broader implications in the areas of social milestones and sexual independence. One mother expressed this by saying

"The minute my daughter was born and I learned about her disability, my first thought was, 'Oh God, I'll never be able to walk her down the aisle.'"

The degree and extent of loss this thought conjures up in the mind of a new (or even an experienced) parent is significant. The discrepancy between the hopes and plans that parents have for their children before a diagnosis of disability and the adaptations that will be required as a result of that diagnosis is repeated and takes on a different face at each new stage of maturity. Additionally, the pain of parents' awareness of their child's limitations and the implications of those limitations for the parents is repeated at each new stage of growth and development.

Denial can help parents for a while, but each reality check and forward step for the child can be a reminder of the initial pain and loss to the parents.

Sometimes the Complexities of the Tasks Are Overwhelming, if Not Impossible

Parents who deal on a daily basis with the difficulties of routine tasks and ordinary decision making may see the complexities of establishing mature relationships as overwhelming or impossible. One parent was able to encapsulate this experience when she said

> "My daughter can't pick out two items of clothes that go together! How in the world is she going to pick out a sensible boyfriend or husband?"

Another parent described his awareness of his child's limitations when he said

> "I've been divorced twice. Picking a good mate is tough enough for all of us who have all our faculties. How can these kids make sense out of choosing a life partner?"

Sexuality Discussions Are Already Difficult Enough

The many reasons why talking about sexuality is so difficult, even with typically developing children, have already been discussed. Now add to those statements the fact that parents will have to go through that talk over and over again. It can be embarrassing for parents, especially if they have not already had this talk with older children and this is their first attempt:

> "I feel so uncomfortable using 'those words.' You know, I'm a single mom and it is so hard talking to a boy about this kind of stuff."

Parents will have to have "that talk" in much more minute detail with their children with intellectual disabilities, and they will probably need the aid of graphic pictures, too. Parents will need to review these facts many, many times with their children to ensure that they remember the information long after the talk is over and that the facts do not get embellished or misinterpreted over time.

> "I'm not sure of the names of all those parts. What if I teach her the wrong ones? Should I use popular slang? Will the other kids laugh if she uses technical terms?"

In explaining and using sexual terminology, there is the extra task of teaching the necessity for discretion and privacy. Parents must communicate that it is OK to talk about these issues—but only in appropriate situations and to appropriate people.

Parents may also be concerned that they are not knowledgeable or experienced enough about sexuality themselves to be the person responsible for their children's sexuality education. They may be unsure how much their child should know or how much they want their child to know.

Parents Have Not Always Decided, in Their Own Minds, What the Goal of This Sexuality Education Is for Their Children

What is the point of all this effort? To many parents of children with intellectual disabilities, it is very hard to decide what the ultimate goal of sexuality education might be. Parents of typically developing children usually have a fairly well-accepted goal: abuse prevention, responsible sexual activity, birth control, and, if desired by their children, a stable, loving marriage (with or without children).

Parents of children with intellectual disabilities cannot always fit their children's goals into such a typical and accepted pattern. A child with an intellectual disability may fit in the pattern at any point along the continuum of social and sexual interaction and stay at that point as part of their ultimate advancement toward independence.

If Parents Ignore Sexuality, Maybe It Will Go Away

The notion that sexuality and sexual interest of an individual with an intellectual disability will disappear if no one acknowledges it is disproven every day. However, the myth that the child "will not know what he or she is missing" persists. Parents sometimes believe or fear that they will create a problem where none exists if they introduce and address sexual issues if their children have not raised the subject directly. One parent said

"Oh my god! I don't think my daughter ever thinks about things like that. She's still playing with Barbie dolls."

The mythology still persists and parents sometimes choose to ignore what is right before their eyes. Hormones undermine parents' desire to deny the existence of sexual development and interest. One father sheepishly admitted

"I was surprised to see my daughter visibly perk up when a boy put his wheelchair next to hers."

Some parents are so uncomfortable with the subject of sex that they are unable to discuss it at all. One mother did not know if her 25-year-old son had ever had any sexuality education in school. Another mother, who stated that her son was an adult who had expressed interest in having a girlfriend, still said that she was hoping that sex would not become an issue. A mother realized the extent of her denial when she said

"I felt so foolish! I thought my son was blowing his nose into his sheets until I realized what was really going on!"

My Child Has Rights, Too

The very basic issue of personal freedom and individual human rights for children and adults with disabilities is brought into sharp focus for parents when it is applied to social and sexual issues. As you would expect, there is no single point of view on this issue.

One father stated his dream for his child with significant multiple disabilities.

"They should legalize sexual surrogacy and prostitution here, like they have in Amsterdam and places in Nevada. That way my boy could enjoy this kind of experience, too. He'll never be able to pass one of these informed consent tests."

The "informed consent test" is an informal reference to a set of standards, different in each state, that interpret each state's laws regarding whether a person has agreed to mutual sexual activity or if a sexual crime has been committed. These standards are used as guidelines to help professionals and law enforcement personnel to determine whether an individual with a disability is competent to make informed choices and decisions regarding sexual activity. These guidelines establish parameters that prevent parents, agency administrators, and potential romantic partners from inadvertently placing a person with a disability in a situation in which he or she may not be able protect him- or herself from sexual victimization.To find the specific information on the laws in any individual state consult the protection and advocacy office in your state. You can find contact information for these offices with any Internet search by state. Or you can search online in the 'Lectric Law Library for the statutes of your state (see http://www.lectlaw.com).

The guidelines are often useful to clarify capacity (i.e., how much the individual understands) and offer legal recourse to prosecute in situations of possible abuse. They help to identify areas in which a person with an intellectual disability may need education, skill building, or other support to strengthen his or her social proficiency as part of a larger long-range life plan.

Sexuality and the law is a very complex and often misunderstood subject. You will find a more detailed discussion of this topic in Chapter 9.

Parents often also have doubts about what their role should be and to what extent they should control their children's decisions in this area of life. As one parent confided

"Is it fair for me to deny my kid a sex life? Am I weird because I hope for this for my son? I'd be really up in arms if my parents tried to deny me that part of life, so how could I do that to my child?"

Some parents are hopeful that their children with intellectual disabilities will have the enjoyment of a long-term loving relationship and a joyful sex life, but they often are unsure about their children's abilities to make mature, sensible decisions.

Other families feel the need to be in greater control of their child's life-altering decisions.

"I don't want to open *that* Pandora's Box! All her life I've always known what's better for her! Why wouldn't I know best about *this*?! And anyway, if there were kids, who'd raise them?"

Parents agonize about how capable their children are to make these very permanent decisions about their own lifestyles. They worry about how a child's poor choices will affect both the child's and their own life trajectory. Parents try to balance their children's abilities with how much personal freedom any one of us is entitled to have, never forgetting the dangers and pleasures of sexual independence. Parents do not always recognize the degree of control that they have had over their children's decisions. Consequently, it is often difficult for parents to think about or accept the idea of their children's personal freedom when it comes to sexual choices, especially if these choices are likely to differ from their own. Parents might be disconcerted if their child with an intellectual disability posed the question to them, "Hey, whose life is it anyway!?"

What if My Child Wants to Have a Child?

No issue is more difficult, causes greater concern, or has more far reaching consequences for the parents of an adult with an intellectual disability than the prospect of their child having a child of his or her own. This issue calls into question the degree to which a parent can or should interfere or approve of the decisions that their adult child may make on a personal level and within the law.

Different families and different cultures have diverse ways in which they are willing and able to support an adult family member with an intellectual disability who wishes to have and raise a child. The authors have known only a very few parents or extended family members of adults with intellectual disabilities who view the prospect of their child having and raising a child as a positive event. Parents need to have the values and resources to apply to this event, or they need to be willing and able to accommodate to it. For some parents, it means becoming grandparents when they thought that would never happen for them. Some people say that it is poverty and the lack of supports, not the disability itself, that make parenthood for adults with intellectual disabilities such a daunting undertaking with very uncertain outcomes.

Most parents of adults with intellectual disabilities with whom we have spoken do not look at a pregnancy, planned or unplanned, as a positive addition to their own or their adult child's life. Scenarios such as 1) a parent or parents with disabilities raising a child with disabilities who may have special needs or 2) a parent or parents with disabilities raising a typically developing child *without a disability* raise potential problems and challenges that are daunting and need deep consideration. A very considerable structure of supports would have to be solidly in place to make a success of either situation.

Many parents acknowledge that their children with disabilities are extremely loving and caring of small children and that, should they have a baby, their baby would experience no lack of affection. Obviously, though, love and affection are not the only qualifications for responsible and comprehensive childrearing.

Parents fear for the future, both the short term and long term, when their children desire to or actually have a child of their own. They fear that even if one or both sets of grandparents and an extended support system can participate in raising this child, and even if there is support from government-sponsored programs or disability or spiritual community groups, this may not be enough to offset what they see as negative effects upon the infant and their own child. Parents may believe that their plans for their own future retirement and economic well-being will be jeopardized by the financial burden that will, most likely, ultimately fall on them. They may also fear that even if a happy marriage produced this new life, that marriage may be endangered by the stresses of caring for a child, especially as the child grows from infancy into the very difficult-to-manage teenage years. Perhaps grandparents will not always be around or healthy enough to participate fully in raising this child.

The solidity and permanence of a strong support system should be assured before an adult with an intellectual disability and his or her parents make a decision of this magnitude. If an adult with an intellectual disability does have a child and it is determined that the parent or parents do not have enough support to safely raise the child, the families, along with social services agencies, may recommend removing the child and placing him or her into foster care and may urge the parents to surrender their parental rights. This would probably be a painful situation for all.

Although it is an extremely controversial subject, parents and care-givers may need to consider the option of termination of pregnancy, by means of abortion, if an unwanted pregnancy occurs. Pregnancy can be the result of consensual sexual activity or rape. Nowadays, the decision to terminate a pregnancy requires the "informed consent" of the pregnant woman, unless she has been deemed "incapable of informed consent" as a result of the evaluation for consent discussed previously in this chapter.

The risk of an unwanted pregnancy is why the subject of birth control, temporary or permanent, should be addressed with individuals with intellectual disabilities who may become sexually active. Parents who advocate abstinence for their children should bear in mind that abstinence provides no protection from a pregnancy resulting from rape. The use of birth control helps avoid the difficult decision between bringing the pregnancy to term (with all of its obvious negative physical and emotional consequences) and ending the pregnancy by means of abortion (with all of its complicated physical, emotional, social, ethical, and even legal repercussions).

Getting Clear Communication from a Child Confounds Parents' Patience

Getting information from a child with an intellectual disability can be very difficult. Unclear and/or inconsistent messages from the child can leave parents in doubt about the things of which they thought they were sure. One parent scratched his head and said:

> "My son claims he is in love with a girl named Elaine, but whenever she calls on the phone, he says, 'Oh no, not her again!'"

Another parent reported that she is not sure what her son and his friends understand about the roles of boyfriends and girlfriends:

> "My son and his friends talk about girls like they're hats. 'If you take A, then I'll take B, and you can have C. But if you want B, then I'll take C, and he can have A.' It never occurs to them that the girls might have something to say about it."

A child's goals or desires may be strongly influenced and shaped by his or her exposure to the media or by fantasy thinking that is not reflective of real insight or thoughtful decision making. Parents need to be attuned to these communication subtleties and need to be able to differentiate between their children's true feelings and those statements and ideas that have been absorbed from other areas of influence. That understanding helps parents respond to the real meaning of their children's communications and not just to the words that are spoken.

> "My daughter moons around about her 'boyfriend.' Turns out the boy is simply a boy in school that she noticed one day. He has no idea who she is or the fact that she considers him her boyfriend. Just believing that she has a boyfriend seems to be enough for her—without any real interaction or understanding of what a boyfriend/girlfriend relationship really is."

Parents Know a Great Deal About Their Children's Activities, Even the Private Ones

With children who have intellectual disabilities, facilitation of social opportunities and transportation can be an issue. The children frequently do not have the capability or the options to arrange their own intimate activities. They usually do not, for example, have the back seat of a car available to them, as many of us did. If they are in the back seat, their parents are probably driving! And that certainly limits their privacy! And, their living arrangements are often under supervision by family or support staff. Consequently, individuals with intellectual disabilities do not have the typical kinds of opportunities for privacy and youthful experimentation.

In gaining access to private sexual opportunities, parents can be put in a very awkward situation—having to arrange dates and meeting times and places, and then transporting the young people to be together.

> "If my son wanted to spend some private time with his girlfriend, I'd have to drive them to some place where they could be alone together and then wait to take him home. I feel like I may as well be getting them a motel room! It is a really weird feeling. Very uncomfortable."
> Another mother said
> "My daughter lives in a group home. She shares her bedroom with another girl. The house has strict rules about not permitting boys upstairs in the bedrooms. How is she ever supposed to develop any kind of intimate relationship?"

The frustration over the difficulty to access appropriate private opportunities for intimacy may sometimes lead individuals with intellectual disabilities to inappropriate behavior, such as choosing inappropriate locations for sexual activity. This can be extremely upsetting for parents and may even have legal repercussions. It is essential for parents to deal with the issue of appropriate places for this kind of expression.

Can/should parents facilitate intimacy by setting up situations in which young people can be together in private? Does this give rise to, condone, or even encourage behavior that the young people might not have initiated on their own? Or, is it helping them to achieve normal expression by filling in the gaps that they cannot do on their own? There are no easy answers here.

There Are Fewer Social Opportunities and More Limited Choices for Possible Relationships

Parents are always concerned about the people with whom their children are involved, even adult children. When the child has an intellectual disability, there is additional concern about the child's understanding, motivation, and functional ability, as well as the social activities and romantic partner or friend that the child chooses. There is often a need for parents of both children to be involved in facilitating with transportation and arrangements. It is important that each child's parents be able to discuss if they are all on the same page about the activities within the relationship and its ultimate goals. Even well-intentioned parents can differ about what is permitted, out of bounds, out of the question, or taboo in a relationship.

> "My daughter wants a boyfriend so badly she would do anything to keep one. She'd be a sitting duck for a guy who even just smiles at her. I'd rather keep her locked up at home than have her taken advantage of by somebody who says he's her boyfriend."
> Another parent asked
> "Where am I going to find a girl for my son? He says he doesn't want to go out with any of the girls from Special Education. He keeps flirting with his job coach, the dental hygienist, and the supermarket checkers where he works. They've all turned him down several times when he's asked them for a date."

As with other areas of socialization, the options available for individuals with intellectual disabilities who want to develop relationships are significantly limited. These individuals generally have access to a smaller number of peers from whom to choose their sweethearts or potential marriage partners than do their age-typical peers. Parents often have to be realistic about the characteristics they would want in their child's partner.

> "My son is crazy about a girl who I think is really awful. He says, 'Mom, she's Playboy enough for me!' Go figure."

While many relationships through the years are likely to be superficial or transitory, it is important for parents to give serious attention to anyone whom the child or young adult expresses sexual interest in beyond a passing attraction.

The degree of control that each parent wishes to have over his or her child's relationships may vary considerably, from total control to laissez faire and anything in between.

Parents—and Children—Have Few Role Models in This Area

The acceptability of sexual expression and fully adult relationships among individuals with intellectual disabilities is a relatively recent area of social inclusion. There are not very many established and successful examples of ongoing relationships for parents to point to as examples for young people to look to for advice or to admire and emulate.

There Are Significant Risks When There Is Sexual Activity with a Partner

The risks associated with sexual activity in the general population are well known: sexually transmitted diseases, unwanted pregnancies, physical injuries, and sexual exploitation or abuse. These same risks are compounded by the presence of an intellectual or developmental disability. Parents need to be confident that their children are knowledgeable about the prevention of sexually transmitted diseases, about birth control, and about the anatomical, biological, and possible psychological implications of sexual activities that involve another person. Again, these can be especially difficult to discuss and they must be reviewed over and over again in detail. This is essential if an individual with an intellectual disability is to be given the autonomy to have sexual relationships.

Obviously, the limitations of the child's cognitive ability may limit the level of understanding that is achievable and must, therefore, be taken into account in determining the amount of autonomy that will be possible. This is an amorphous concept, which may fluctuate and may be difficult to assess, but which must be taken into consideration at every step along the way.

The same applies to the awareness of and prevention of sexual exploitation and abuse in sexual relationships. Children and adults with intellectual disabilities tend to be less critical and less skeptical about the motives of others. They will be more vulnerable to exploitation unless they are painstakingly and frequently instructed in discerning the motives of others' actions. Having information about exploitation, however, does not guarantee that a person with an intellectual disability will recognize an abusive relationship or that the individual will call upon that information and use it when he or she does recognize an abusive situation. Parents often teach their children to be cooperative and docile for much of their lives and to follow the instructions of authority figures.

Safety in private situations often requires assertiveness and resistance to the requests and pressures of others, the opposite of what usually has already been internalized. Parents need to keep the lines of communication open with their children even after they have earned sexual autonomy.

> "A girl in our neighborhood thought she had a boyfriend and said she was engaged to him. This so-called boyfriend was playing her along in order to get into her apartment, have sex with her, and steal her stuff."

There are risks associated with sexual activity regardless of who is engaging in the behavior or what intellectual ability or disability may exist! There are great joys and benefits to having a social and sexual life as well. Parents must accept the notion that all activity carries risk. When parents give their children with intellectual disabilities the tools to manage the risks and maximize the safety of social and sexual activities, they are giving them a gift. Parents help their children when they replace fear and guilt with education and support to build a quality life experience.

WHAT PARENTS CAN DO

It is important for parents to have an accurate and fully dimensional assessment of their children. Parents' portraits of their children can sometimes be colored by the great love that they have for them. This can often make parents overly protective, treating their children as if they were much younger. Conversely, this great love can sometimes lead to an overly positive perception and cause parents to treat their children as more capable than they really are. It is important for parents to try to set aside their fears and fantasies and develop a realistic evaluation of their children, especially related to social and sexual development issues.

Parents can ask their children's teacher or counselor to help form this realistic picture. Counselors have formal evaluations that they can use to interpret a child's behaviors. Teachers observe the child every day interacting with other children, responding to personal responsibilities, and managing the demands of the school environment in the classroom, on the playground, and in the cafeteria.

Parents need to remember that the impact of an intellectual disability is usually unevenly expressed in the different aspects of a child's development and achievement. Academic progress may not parallel social maturity; self control may be more affected by the disability than speech development; biological maturity may arrive at a typical age, but emotional adulthood may come later.

Parents should think about how to support their children to make changes from childish or silly behaviors to more mature ones. Helping a child learn how to express his or her wishes is essential and can help avoid an adversarial relationship between concerned parents and their child. It may take some more time in the short run but be well worth it in the long run to get the child used to participating in negotiation and decision making at available opportunities.

Parents can start by helping their children make choices and compromises about recreation, food, or clothing. Parents should find out what their child wants and ask assistance from the child to achieve that goal. Later, when there is need for negotiation about issues concerning socialization or sexual activity, the child will have experiences from which to draw and can be an active participant in the discussion. If there are no available opportunities, parents can create some!

The media, such as TV, movies, music, and teen magazines, can have an enormous influence on what children learn about the world beyond their school and family lives. Adults typically know that life is not portrayed realistically in the media. Individuals with intellectual disabilities, however, may not understand that this is so. To address this, parents can sit down with their children and watch a few TV shows that their children watch. Parents can then use this relaxed leisure time to create "teachable moments," in which they can find out the children's understanding of the show's story line, the characterizations, and the implicit messages in the program. Parents can take advantage of the time together to discuss issues raised by the TV show within the context of their family's value system, ethical code, and cultural traditions.

As with any of the children in a family, a child with an intellectual disability may ultimately adopt many of the family's closely held beliefs, but perhaps not all of them. It's important that a child with an intellectual disability has the same opportunity as any other member of the family to reflect upon those personal values for him- or herself.

Parents can also make use of situations that arise in daily life and add to a child's knowledge base about social and sexual development issues: observing a couple kissing in the park or a pregnant woman at the movie theater, walking through the underwear department at the clothing store, or discussing an upcoming wedding or a new baby in the family. These can all be opportunities to address aspects of sexuality education in a natural and informal way.

In addition, it is important for parents not to overreact when their children bring up a sexual subject that makes them uncomfortable. If necessary, parents can say that it is a little hard for them to talk about that subject, but that they will try. Parents should attempt to be responsive and address their children's questions at the time that they are raised. It is important that parents communicate to their children that sexual subjects are not "off-limits" and convey the comforting feeling that they are approachable about anything and everything that may be on their children's minds. If a parent is so uncomfortable that he or she simply cannot talk about sex, the parent should enlist the help of a trusted adult family member or friend to help carry out the discussions as necessary. Professionals with expertise and experience can assist in making both parent and child more comfortable and can advise about specifics related to sexuality education.

Often, parents can anticipate many of the questions that their child might ask and can prepare for them in advance. One option is for parents to go to a local bookstore or library and get a book that provides information to parents about sexuality. Parents can tailor that information to the age and cognitive ability of his or her child. Being informed can give parents confidence to try to be the resource to answer questions fully and accurately.

If a child does not bring up sexual issues or questions on his or her own, parents should use their judgment and find an opportunity to bring up certain subjects. For example, a rumor that a celebrity is said to be pregnant can generate a question such as "How do you think things will change for her now that she's going to be a mom?" An invitation to a family wedding can generate a questions such as "What does it take to be a good wife or husband?" or "Can you tell why Jennifer and Glenn love each other and are so good for each other?" or "What are some good qualities that you would look for in a boyfriend/girlfriend?" A newspaper headline that reports catching a rapist can generate questions such as "What does the word 'rape' mean?" or "Who should a person tell if he or she is raped?" Even a trip to the pharmacy to buy feminine hygiene supplies can generate discussions such as, "There are so many different kinds of sanitary pads. Let's check them out and see how they are different from each other,"or "You don't need these pads just yet, but when you get a little more grown up you will get a period just like Mom. What do you think are some signs that a girl is growing up?" or "Now that you've gotten your period, there are some other things that will change, too. Let's talk about these changes."

There is great benefit for parents to have a formal or informal association with other parents of children and adults with intellectual disabilities. They can discuss issues that they share, exchange helpful information about community resources and events, tell about techniques that have been successful for them in similar situations with their children, and suggest advocacy strategies. More importantly, they can air their hopes and fears and appreciate the successes of each other's children from the perspective that only another parent of a child with an intellectual disability can have.

It is important for parents to help their children envision a realistic future with regard to sexual maturity. This should not only include the parents' personal values but should also seek to develop the values of their children, which may not be identical to their own. Discussions about potential parenthood should not simply reflect the media version of relationships or the unreality of the "Gerber baby" version of parenthood.

If parenthood is not a likely benefit to an individual with an intellectual disability, family members can gradually show the advantages and express the values of being "child free." It is appropriate to comment on incidents that illuminate the difficulties of raising children, such as observing a parent having trouble with an unruly child in the supermarket. Being an aunt or uncle can be a practical, pleasing, and gratifying arrangement for married or single adults with intellectual disabilities: a lot of the love and a lot less of the responsibility.

Once a sexually active adult with an intellectual disability has decided that parenthood would make his or her life too difficult or that it is not the lifestyle that he or she is interested in leading, the arrangements for long-term or permanent birth control can be addressed. Although sterilization of individuals with intellectual disabilities conjures up hideous images of a long history of past abuses, vasectomy or tubal ligation is a choice that many individuals with intellectual limitations are capable of making with support. They are often relieved to be able to put the responsibilities of birth control out of their sexual relationship. Education that uses ability-appropriate materials to discuss and evaluate the risks and benefits of various options can assist a person with an intellectual disability make an informed decision that reflects his or her own wishes.

CONCLUSION

Clearly, parents and children with intellectual disabilities have an important investment in decisions about sexuality education and expression. There is a wide variation of opinion and ability on the part of parents and children to effectively cope with this subject. There is not simply one right answer, but rather there are many right *questions*. Ultimately, caring parents and their children will make the effort required to come to terms with the extent and the ways in which sexuality can be incorporated successfully into their lives.

REFERENCES

Bellafante, G. (2005, June 5). Fact of life, for their eyes only. *The New York Times*, pp. F1, F4.

A Summary of Guidelines for Parents as Sexuality Educators

No one expects a parent to suddenly be an expert sexuality educator for their child with a developmental or intellectual disability after reading a chapter such as this one. In spite of that, PARENTS DO HAVE A VERY IMPORTANT ROLE!

Here are some guidelines that are helpful for parents:

1. Be aware that you are a very important role model to your child. Make sure you demonstrate honesty, respect, and appropriateness in relationships with the people you know and support, especially when your child is present. Use the CIRCLES® model as a guide if you are doubtful of how to act.

2. Work hard to assure that your child knows that it is always safe to discuss any personal issues with you without fear of criticism or judgment.

3. Team up with teachers and other professionals to develop a realistic plan for your child's social as well as educational, vocational, and residential future. Make sure that social and recreational planning is included in any other plan created for your child.

4. Assist your child with intellectual disabilities to know about and participate in a variety of community and disability specialized social experiences.

The registered trademark CIRCLES® and the descriptive material herein drawn from copyrighted material published in The CIRCLES® Series are used with the permission of James Stanfield Company. All rights reserved. Duplication in any form is prohibited. For information about the CIRCLES® Video Series, contact James Stanfield Publishing Company, 800-421-6534.

5. Support good social interactions that you see your child having by complimenting your child and by facilitating similar events or interactions.

6. Help your child to access sexuality education and services in your community. Use meaningful sexuality education programs that go beyond simply naming body parts and personal hygiene.

7. Learn more about sexuality and about developmental and intellectual disabilities by taking a look at items in the bibliography at the end of the book. Use your public library and reliable Internet resources.

8. Familiarize yourself with the signs of sexual abuse and know what actions to take if you suspect sexual abuse.

9. Use "teachable moments" to help your child understand and manage sexual interest and expression in ways that are socially acceptable.

10. Make sure that your child understands what is private and what is public behavior.

11. Suggest a "Social Development and Sexuality" category in the annual review, individualized education program, individualized service plan, or other team meeting process.

12. Do not hesitate to seek out professional help or advice if needed.

AND ABOVE ALL...

13. Show respect for your child's sexuality as he or she develops toward becoming a participating adult, having a full and satisfying life.

5

Social Support Systems for Quality Service Delivery

A Historical View

Amy Gerowitz

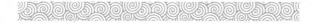

The world of supports and services for people with intellectual disabilities is changing. People with disabilities, their families, friends, and those who work most closely with them are asking for, indeed demanding, education, work, homes, recreation, and social and intimate relationships in the community. Most people with intellectual disabilities and those who care about them want full inclusion, and efforts are underway to make this happen. This chapter outlines the evolution of attitudes toward people with intellectual disabilities and the impact of those attitudes on available services, supports, and relationships. This evolution, however, has not occurred in a linear progression. Many of the attitudes and service configurations discussed in this chapter as ideas of the past are still quite prevalent. However, many more people with intellectual disabilities are experiencing increased opportunities for independence, inclusion, sexual expression, and relationships. They also are experiencing increased community participation as society begins to accept them as individual people capable of and entitled to live the fullest life possible. This chapter also provides a framework for understanding the contemporary support system for people with intellectual disabilities.

The attitudes that drove the initial development of services and supports for people with disabilities were those of separateness and segregation. The thinking was that people with disabling conditions, once known as "the feeble minded," needed separation and protection from society and that society needed separateness and protection from people with disabilities. This resulted in a system that caused people with disabilities to:

- Be in "special, separate" systems
- Be in relationships with people like themselves
- Be in large congregate facilities, sheltered workshops, separate schools, and segregated social activities
- Be sent away to treatment facilities for care and training
- Be placed in residential programs
- Be prevented from having intimate or sexual relationships
- Have others say what kinds of services they needed
- Have others decide what was good for them, what they needed, and what they should want

As you read this chapter, you will learn about the effect of attitudes toward people with disabilities and how these attitudes affected services they received and their rights to express themselves in personal relationships.

PART 1: HISTORY

The history of supports and services for people with intellectual and other disabilities reflects the attitudes that drove separation, exclusion, and the development of institutions. As attitudes changed, the configuration of supports, public policy, and societal acceptance led to more inclusive open environments and services.

Segregation

The prevailing wisdom of the late nineteenth and first half of the twentieth century in the United States was that people with disabilities would benefit from separation from their community and families. Well-intentioned reformers, physicians, and policy makers called them eternal children who were "gifts from God" and "special people" to be cared for. Those paid staff members who worked with individuals with disabilities were considered "special," and made all of the decisions for those that depended on them. In fact, few in society thought of people with disabilities as being capable of expressing opinions and preferences or making choices about where to live and how to spend their time. Individuals with disabilities were not asked what they wanted; they were typically sent away and often forgotten. Physicians often advised families when their children were born with disabilities that they could not possibly care for their child at home and that it would be best to send the child away to an institution. In some cases parents were told to forget that they ever had the child. In many cases, younger children were never told about the existence of an older sibling who had been institutionalized. It is difficult to imagine a mother and father being told that the best thing they can do is to forget their child. How families reacted to this advice provides an interesting examination of the service system during this time. Read what happened when Maurice found out about a brother he didn't know he had. Later you will meet other families who ignored the professional advice and you will see how that affected family relationships and life.

David lived in a large community facility that provided residential and training services to 80 people with very severe physical and cognitive disabilities. David, like most of the people who lived there, had previously lived in a state-operated institution for the mentally retarded. David's records showed no involved family, and he had a state appointed guardian. One day, a 25-year-old man named Maurice visited the residential facility. He had just found out that David was his twin brother and had been sent to an institution in the northern part of the state as a young child. Maurice always thought that he was an only child. When his parents died and Maurice went through the household papers, he was devastated to find that he had an unknown twin brother who had profound disabilities. No one from the family had ever visited or contacted David until the day of Maurice's visit at age 25. This was the first time Maurice and David had ever met.

When Maurice and David were born, it is likely, indeed probable, that their parents were given the advice that led to the separation of these twins. Imagine Maurice's shock on that day in 1985 when he discovered that he had a brother he had never even known about! Imagine what it did to these parents to make this decision and live with this secret for 25 years!

Maurice visited David a few times, but had difficulty connecting with his brother. After awhile he stopped visiting and moved to another city. They just could not overcome the 25 years of separation, so each man was left without family.

Institutions

Institutions for individuals with disabilities were developed as self-contained microcosms of the world. They had, for example, schools, hospitals, cemeteries, farms, greenhouses, and cottages or wards that housed the people who lived there. As residents with disabilities grew to adulthood, they would often work on the grounds of the institution. Almost no one had the opportunity to engage in relationships, hold hands, date, kiss, or marry. In fact these behaviors were strongly discouraged. Residents typically spent their days inside cottages or sometimes in day activity centers or sheltered workshops. Although these institutions were designated for "the mentally retarded," some people were placed there because they were classified as slow learners, had seizure disorders, were physically limited, misbehaved in school, were indigent, or even because their parents had died and there was nothing else to do with them. The residents at these institutions knew no other life and often became quite efficient in the work they were assigned.

There were no federal laws mandating the education of children with disabilities until the early 1970s. As a result most of these children received almost no or at best a very limited education. You will have the opportunity to read more about the effect of mandatory education later in this chapter.

The staff members and the residents of these institutions became their own self-contained communities. Many well-meaning people worked and volunteered at such institutions, thinking that institutions were the best things for these "special people." The idea of people with disabilities needing or wanting companionship, relationships, or sexual expression was never considered. People spent their lives hidden from the typical pressures and delights of society, including love and companionship. While there were forward thinking people earlier, it was probably not until the later 1980s that the more prevalent view was that people with disabilities were entitled to share in this full expression of life. In large part this was a result of changing attitudes and societal expectations and mores that ultimately led to changes in public policy and service delivery.

Changing Attitudes

The 1960s ushered in a decade of significant social change: the war in Vietnam, the civil rights and women's rights movements, and the sexual revolution profoundly altered the way our society treated people. Rosa Parks would not sit in the back of the bus because she was black; women demanded equal rights and accessible birth control. In addition to the legalization of abortion in the United States in 1973, attitudes changed toward relationships and sexual expression. Society's traditional values and mores were all open to question. The field of separate, segregated services for citizens with disabilities did not escape this scrutiny.

In 1966, Robert Kennedy visited Willowbrook State School in Staten Island, New York. He declared that Willowbrook "was not fit for even animals to live in" (Schlesinger, 1978, p. 679). As a result of Senator Kennedy's series of unannounced visits to Willowbrook, news of the conditions there became even more widespread. Children, Robert Kennedy said, "just rock back and forth. They grunt and gibber and soil themselves...there are no civil liberties for those put in the cells of Willowbrook—living amidst brutality, human excrement, and intestinal disease"(Schlesinger, 1978, p. 679).

In the early 1970s, several books were published that exposed the world to what was happening in institutions. The institutions were described as "hell on earth" (Burton and Kaplan, 1974). In 1972, Geraldo Rivera, then a young television reporter, was able to get inside one of these institutions, Willowbrook State School in Staten Island, New York, with hidden cameras. Through a series of televised news reports, he showed the world the abuse and neglect he found there.

Unfortunately, Willowbrook was not an isolated example of the results of segregation and separation. However, Willowbrook came to symbolize everything that was wrong with the care of people with intellectual disabilities (Duggar, 1993). The United States Department of Justice, families, and other local, state, and federal governmental groups began to place institutions under much greater scrutiny. Families resisted sending their children away and began to demand high-quality services in the community.

Alternatives for funding, service provision, and monitoring were discussed and developed. With changing attitudes came changed public programs. Institutions were no longer hidden backwaters minimally overseen by state and local governments. As the public became aware of conditions for people with disabilities, there was a demand for greater oversight and protection and for a broader array of places for people with disabilities to live.

Changing Public Policy

A series of public policy initiatives in the early 1970s helped move society forward in its treatment of people with disabilities. The Rehabilitation Act of 1973 (PL 93-112) was the first civil rights legislation to prohibit discrimination against people with disabilities. Organizations receiving federal funding could not discriminate based on a person's disability and had to make reasonable accommodation for people with disabilities. The Education for All Handicapped Children Act of 1975 (PL 94-142), which later became the Individuals with Disabilities Education Act (IDEA) of 1990 (PL 101-476), required public schools to make available a free and appropriate public education to all eligible children with disabilities. These laws represented a significant change in the opportu-

nities for people with disabilities. Policy makers and society were beginning to recognize that all people have the right to live and learn, develop relationships, and become integral parts of society.

Various state and federal programs began to pay for and regulate
the care of those with disabilities living in institutions. Efforts began to
improve living conditions, help people move back to their communities,
provide education for children, and help families make different kinds
of decisions for their children.

Medicaid is a federal/state matching program that provides for
health care, preventative services, and institutional and home and community supports. In 1974 the Medicaid program expanded its scope
beyond health care for the poor and elderly and developed a special
classification in long-term care for facilities providing residential services to people with intellectual disabilities: the Intermediate Care Facility for the Mentally Retarded (ICF/MR). Society at large was learning
that people with disabilities were capable of intellectual growth and
change. Shutting individuals away in institutions that did little more
than assure that they were fed and had a place to sleep was no longer
acceptable.

Following the enactment of these laws and programs, significant
federal funds were sent to states. Institutions were updated and mod-
ernized. Wards housing 10 to 20 people were replaced with single rooms
for two to four people, privacy in bathing and showering was required,
and people received training and education. Community residential
facilities such as group homes and independent apartments were developed in greater numbers. However, the prevailing attitudes that developed these models still reflected the underlying premise that people
with disabilities could not decide things for themselves. Consequently
the service structures were hierarchical, developmental, and medical.

For example, people with disabilities were identified as to the
extent of their disabilities. It was not uncommon, for example, to hear
terminology referring to people with disabilities as the "profounds," the
"non-ams," the "behaviors," and the "feeds." To counter the many years
in which people in institutions had done absolutely nothing, the concept of *active treatment* (Code of Federal Regulations [CFR], 483.440) was
created, and residents were rigorously "programmed" or trained all day
long. This meant that schedules were developed that required that people be engaged constantly. Staff would often set up games that people
couldn't or didn't way to play, rolling balls back and forth, basically trying to make everyone look busy. Sex education, if addressed at all, usually only covered putting makeup on women and teaching men how to
dress better. Table 5.1 outlines the philosophy of this model of training
and how it evolved over time.

Table 5.1. The evolution in services and supports

Focal question	Era of institutions	Era of deinstitution- alization	Era of community membership
Who is the person of concern?	The patient	The client	The citizen
What is the typical setting?	An institution	A group home, work- shop, special school, or class- room	A person's home, local business, the neighborhood school
How are the services organized?	In facilities	In a continuum of options	A unique array of supports tailored to the individual
What is the model?	Custodial/medical	Developmental/ behavioral	Individual support
What are the services?	Care	Programs	Supports
How are services planned?	Through a plan of care	Through an individu- alized habilitation plan	Through a person- centered plan
Who controls the decision?	A professional (usually an MD)	An interdisciplinary team	The individual
What is the planning context?	Standards of pro- fessional prac- tice	Team consensus	A circle of support
What has the highest priority?	Basic needs	Skill development, behavior manage- ment	Self-determination and relationships
What is the objective?	Control or cure	To change behavior	To change the envi- ronment/attitudes

From Knoll, J. (1992). From community-based alternatives to inclusion communities. *In Inclusive Communities, 1,* 9. Adapted with permission.

In addition, plans of care, previously developed by physicians and nurses at the institutions, were developed by interdisciplinary teams, including therapists, clinicians, and other professionals. While the inclusion of an interdisciplinary team was a step forward, the team of professionals decided everything about the person's life, and the person with the disability and his or her family were still left out of the decision making. Front line workers, families, and individuals themselves sat in on planning meetings, only to listen as professionals described the individual's deficits, read assessments filled with complex medical terminology, and established clinical goals. Then, at the end of the meeting, the facilitator would turn to the parent and ask, "Do you have anything to add?" After years of being told that the professionals knew best, few parents or guardians had the courage to add anything, and very few had the confidence or training to challenge these professionals with questions. While the regulations mandated that people with disabilities sit in on their team meetings, often people with the most profound disabilities could be found sleeping or tearing magazine pages as they sat through the meetings. These meetings regularly dragged on for hours, as clinicians read lengthy reports, and hardly anyone paid attention. Often people came into the meeting read their report and quickly left. Incidents such as these happened over and over again and, unfortunately, are still occurring today. The same mode of team planning often occurred in schools as well.

> Arthur lived in a state institution for most of his life. He had both intellectual and physical disabilities. Arthur did not know how to masturbate with his hands, but he knew he liked how it felt to have his penis stimulated, so he would often lie down on the floor and push hard to stimulate himself. He would often wander the halls of the institution and stimulate himself. When the team met to discuss what Arthur should be doing, much of the time was spent trying to provide him with alternative activities so that he wouldn't want to masturbate. Staff members stopped Arthur whenever he was caught stimulating himself and directed him to another activity.
>
> As you read this chapter, think about how Arthur might have been supported differently if people thought about what he wanted in his life.

Relationships and sexuality were rarely discussed, although there was an ICF/MR regulation that required that the interdisciplinary team address and develop programs for social development including the formation of "maintaining appropriate roles and fulfilling relationships with others" (CFR 483.440 c [3] [v]). This was one of the first times that a regulation required that service providers consider the forming of relationships for people with disabilities.

Deinstitutionalization

Deinstitutionalization, moving people with intellectual and multiple disabilities out of separate state institutions and into the community, resulted in the development of a network of community residential supports and services. This movement began in earnest in the early 1980s and it is still ongoing today. In most cases, people with disabilities moved back with their families or into their own home (usually a group home, a small shared apartment, or a large congregate facility housing many people). The concept of a continuum of care was developed early on in the deinstitutionalization movement. This meant that people with disabilities who wanted to live in the community should move from larger, more segregated settings to smaller, more inclusive settings based on their skill development and increased independence. Eligibility criteria to "graduate" to greater independence and readiness skills were identified. For example, a person might have to prove that he or she can cook simple meals, do laundry, count change, or get along well with others. These criteria, however, effectively excluded some people from ever being able to graduate to a new level of living. The same concepts to determine a young child's reading readiness in preschool and kindergarten were often applied to adults with intellectual disabilities. That is, if a person did not move through the expected continuum of skills, the person could become stuck in a more restrictive setting, even if he or she wanted to live in a smaller home with fewer people. For example, a person with challenging behaviors who would become more upset around a lot of people could not move out of a larger congregate facility and into his or her own place until his or her behavior improved. The behavior was unlikely to improve, however, if the person had to continue to living in the same situation. The continuum-of-care concept kept many people frozen in place. The continuum looked like this:

State Institution → Large Community ICF/MR → Group Home → Supported Living

People with disabilities essentially could become stuck in the system, often having arrived there for reasons other than those having to do with a disability.

As late as 1990, a colleague of mine was visiting a state-operated institution. This place was reputed to be state of the art, certified, accredited, and well-funded—the showcase institution in that state. Her observations of the place did not support its reputation. In one cottage where several people lived, a 15-year-old African American girl named Janet came up and started talking with my colleague. My colleague saw no visible sign of intellectual or physical disability. After chatting with Janet, my colleague asked her guides why Janet was living at this institution, a place reported to be serving those with the most profound and severe cognitive and physical disabilities. "Oh," they said, "the judge in the small town nearby had ordered her there because she was incorrigible." "Incorrigible" appeared to mean "sexually promiscuous."

My colleague was quite shocked, but went on her way. About six months later, she returned. She entered a building, and Janet approached her again and greeted her by name. My colleague learned that the judge had barred Janet from leaving the institution and even attending public high school in the community because she had been sexually active. She was essentially imprisoned in this system with no right of appeal. My colleague was told later that Janet had been transferred to a group home for people with the dual diagnosis of mental illness and mental retardation. In 1990, a judge in a small town could still order a girl to be segregated from her community and placed in an institution as a punishment.

The philosophy of the continuum lost acceptance over time as people began to accept individuals with disabilities as people and learned that it was possible and in fact most desirable to help these individuals create a life with the supports they needed. So instead of passing through a continuum of care (which some people could never do), people with disabilities could move on. The concept of readiness was replaced with that of support (see Table 5.1) so that people no longer had to acquire a specific set of skills to:

- Live in the community
- Go to a public school
- Go to the sheltered workshop
- Go to a real job
- Go on community outings
- Have friends
- Learn about sex and intimacy
- Have a real relationship

Change was also occurring in other parts of the community. As a direct result of the Individuals with Disabilities Education Act (IDEA) in 1990, children with disabilities began to be educated within their communities. Prior to 1975, communities often had separate, segregated schools for children with disabilities, which often only those labeled as "high functioning" could attend. Children with challenging behaviors, physical limitations, and lower cognitive abilities typically were kept at home. Once education became mandatory, however, many states and local school districts expanded the number of schools or established separate schools for children with intellectual and other developmental disabilities. For those considered "too disabled" to go to school, the requirement was that they received 1 hour per day of home training. There was only minimal respite care, and families often struggled to gain the most basic services and supports.

Families and advocates fought for the rights of their children with disabilities to be included in the public school system. Like other civil rights pioneers, these children and their families faced exclusion and rejection, but they led the way for others to more fully participate in community life. The evolution of services for children in schools followed the pattern of services discussed earlier in this chapter, from the professionals deciding everything to the increased involvement of the student and his or her family.

PART 2: LIFE IN THE COMMUNITY

In a follow-up article on conditions at Willowbrook, *The New York Times* reported that the former residents now cook, shop, and marry the people they love. People with disabilities, their families, and their advocates no longer wanted or would accept separate lives. This section will explore the impact of that change.

Living and Learning in the Community

During the 1980s, advocates, self-advocates, family members, and professionals urged more vigorously that society create support systems that would help people with disabilities live the life that they wanted, not one dictated by a team of professionals. More and more families insisted on keeping their children at home. Families who had rejected the advice of doctors in the 1960s and 1970s paved the way for families horrified at the idea of sending their children away. Sometimes it worked out well, sometimes it didn't. Here are two families' experiences. One of these families' experiences is my own personal story:

> A family in Pennsylvania gave birth to a son, Joe, with Down syndrome in 1965. As the mother and father sat in the doctor's office trying to figure out what to do, the doctor said that they should send Joe to an institution. Neither parent could fathom sending their son away. As they walked out of the office, they agreed that they would find a way to keep Joe at home. They did, and today, while Joe has trouble expressing himself, he has become part of the community. He works in a laundry facility, has friends, and is an integral part of his family. This family, like thousands of others, had to figure it out for themselves.
>
> When I lived in a northeastern state in the early 1970s, the family across the street had many children. They were a large family, and their children went to school down the street. Each morning I saw the children walking to school; however, one child remained in the house looking out the window. Day or evening, this girl with intellectual and physical disabilities looked out the window. Her family opted to keep her home, but there were probably very limited services available for her, and her family was either unaware or unwilling to use them. For the three years I lived in that house, whenever I looked over, I would see the girl looking out the window.

In order for families to keep their children at home, they had to figure things out for themselves. Policy and funding only supported institutions and services away from home. However, as attitudes began to change, so did funding; the structure and funding of services for people

Table 5.2. Changes in where people with disabilities lived and how money was spent from 1977 to 2002

	1977	2002
State-operated institutions	149,892 people	44,242 people
Settings with fewer than six people	20,000 people	298,375 people
Public spending	$9.8 billion	$34.6 billion

From Braddock, D., Hemp, R., & Rizzolo, M.C. (2004). State of the States in developmental disabilities: 2004. *Mental Retardation, 42*(5), 356–370. Adapted with permission.

with disabilities began to support more community involvement. Table 5.2 summarizes the changes in where people lived and how money was spent. In 1977, 149,892 people with disabilities lived in state-operated institutions for individuals with mental retardation, whereas in 2002 that number was reduced to 44,242. Along with that change was a change in the types of places people lived. For instance, 20,000 people with disabilities lived in homes with fewer than six people in 1977; this number jumped to 298,375 in 2002. Additionally, public spending increased from $9.8 billion in 1977 to $34.6 billion in 2002 (Braddock, Hemp, & Rizzolo, 2004).

The Medicaid Home and Community Based Waiver was developed as a non-institutional option for Medicaid dollars, and states put money into supported living programs, which allowed people with disabilities to live in smaller settings in their own communities. Stringent regulations around activities and the planning process were replaced with systems designed to focus on the person and the life he or she was living and how that compared to the life he or she wanted to live.

The Changing Philosophy of Supports: Person-Centered and Individualized Supports

Slowly, the thinking of people with disabilities, family members, advocates, private providers of services and public policy makers shifted from habilitation to support, from developmental steps to choice, from graduating through a continuum to figuring out how to help a person get the life that person wanted. New strategies, such as personal futures planning and person-centered planning, were created to look at each person's strengths and challenges in addition to his or her long- and short-term dreams and aspirations to determine how to create and nurture opportunities for full community participation.

Person-Centered Planning

Person-centered planning reflects a shift in thinking about the field of developmental disabilities, changing the focus from "program-oriented, formulaic models of care to individually tailored supports based on individual choices and preferences" (Taub, Smith, & Bradley, 2003). It focuses on people's strengths and preferences, not what is wrong with them, and what they actually want to do. While person-centered planning requires that professionals honor a person's choice, it still also requires that professionals help the person develop a life that is both healthy and safe (Smull, 2003). We will explore this further later in this chapter.

Self-determination, self-advocacy, community inclusion, and real choices are the critical determinants in person-centered planning. The model that was built around the formal interdisciplinary team was replaced by a model consisting of a team with members who knew the person and, in many cases, had been specifically selected by the person and/or his or her closest advocates. Formal meetings in conference rooms were replaced or supplemented with small meetings in coffee shops and people's homes. In these smaller, more intimate settings, people could focus on what was actually important for the person. Large groups of strangers were not discussing the most intimate details of someone's life. As a result of this new model, clinicians and therapists can apply their expertise in ways that assist the person toward achieving his or her desired lifestyle, personal goals, and future.

Typically, people living in the general population are anxious to develop intimate and personal relationships, or they are in great threat of isolation and loneliness. People with disabilities, however, often received little or no information about human sexuality, even about what was happening to their own bodies. Effective and individualized person-centered planning can help people with disabilities lead more fulfilling and informed lives and overcome some of the fears that come with ignorance and misinformation.

> Althea is 29 years old and lives in a complex where people who are quite independent have their own apartments. Each person is provided with needed supports by a residential provider agency. Althea uses a wheelchair and works in the community. She has a history of reported sexual and physical abuse—her uncle had sex with her when she was a child and told her he'd kill her family if she told anybody—and her parents have been in and out of the legal and social welfare systems.
>
> Growing up, Althea was never given any information about sex, her body, or what to expect as she went through puberty. "When I first started my period, I thought I was dying. The therapist at school helped me." She went on to report that her father cried and her grandmother "filled me in on a few the details" of puberty. Her friends and boyfriends taught her about sex.
>
> Althea became sexually active when she was 20 and chose to use the birth control pill so she would not become pregnant. Now, her person-centered planning team is helping to support her to make good decisions about relationships and sex.

Loneliness and the craving for friends and relationships is something that must be addressed through person-centered planning and system change if people are to experience fully involved, satisfying lives. Programs throughout the country are working to help people with disabilities develop interests, opportunities, and relationships that may help them connect more with their communities. Some have dating services, others have couples' groups, and still others have general interest groups.

John O'Brien and Connie Lyle O'Brien developed much of the thinking about person-centered planning. The five major accomplishments in person-centered planning that guide the development of an individual's personal vision include:

- Community presence: How can we increase the presence of a person in local community life?

- Community participation: How can we expand and deepen a person's friendships?

- Dignity: How can we enhance the reputation a person has and increase the number of valued ways a person can contribute?

- Promoting choice: How can we help a person have more control and choice in his or her life?

- Supporting contribution: How can we assist a person to develop more competencies? (O'Brien & O'Brien, 1992)

How does person-centered planning translate into the real lives of people who live in all kinds of places and experience a range of challenges, opportunities, and backgrounds?

The following three stories provide an opportunity for reflection on the importance of focusing on the individual and his or her whole life.

Around 1990, Betty, a 34-year-old woman with cerebral palsy and moderate intellectual disabilities, lived in a community residential facility providing services to 52 people with severe and profound physical and cognitive disabilities. Prior to living there, she had resided in a state institution. Although her current home was large, it was considered to be relatively advanced in thinking about people first. One day, while Betty was at the sheltered workshop, she met Steve, a man with intellectual disabilities and cerebral palsy, and they developed a relationship. They fell in love. Steve lived at home with his parents and as a result of his cerebral palsy had an awkward gait and limited use of his arms. He visited Betty often, and she was invited to his home often. Shortly thereafter, Betty went to see her caseworker and said that she and Steve wanted to have intimate sexual relations. The interdisciplinary team all discussed Betty's declaration. They were not shocked or appalled at the idea of this increased intimacy, but they did not know how to help Betty and Steve plan. They scheduled a meeting with Steve's parents. His parents informed the team that Steve was physically incapable of having sex, so the matter was dropped.

When the team met again, they developed strategies and plans to help Betty and Steve have some time in private, and that was as far as it went.

The facility team spoke with the county case manager about the possibility of Betty moving into her own apartment in the community. Unfortunately, however, the county case manager assured the team that there were no funds for this. Since Betty had a place to live, she could be on the waiting list, but an apartment for Betty was not a priority.

An alternative solution: If the philosophy underlying person-centered planning and individualized supports had been in place at the time, many things could have been different for Betty. Since her relationship with Steve was the most important thing in her life at the time, the team could have focused on how to help them nurture that relationship. They could have suggested gaining more information about Steve's reported physical limitations and discussed the options for sex education and medical treatment with Betty and Steve. Even more importantly, the team could have focused and worked harder with the county case manager to find a way for Betty to have her own place or to at least live with fewer than 51 other people, or possibly have her own room. The facilitator could have sat quietly with Betty and discussed what was most important to her. Maybe the whole team, not to mention everyone who worked at the place, would not have been informed of the details of Betty's most intimate life. The objective could have been helping Betty get the life she wanted, not to just fitting in with the rules and structures of the service delivery system.

Adam is 26 years old and has cerebral palsy and a rare endocrine condition. Until recently, he lived with his family in a northeast suburban community. Adam weighed 2 pounds at birth and had several surgeries before he was 8 months old, and doctors did not expect him to survive. One doctor said, "We could not do the work we need to do, if we contemplated the quality of life." Adam survived his surgeries. His parents advocated for the best possible services for him. Adam participated in both segregated and inclusive classes, and he developed acquaintances but did not find real friends or relationships outside of his family.

Adam was affectionate; his father described him as a "breast man." Adam often touched women's breasts, and his family realized that this unacceptable behavior would further exclude him from opportunities in typical society. Through community networking they retained a professional to provide Adam with sex education and teach him strategies and cues related to developing more appropriate behaviors.

His father said that what they did for Adam was no different than send-ing a debutante to charm school. The sex educator became part of his IEP team. This story is an example of person-centered planning at work: in order to help Adam develop the life he wanted, those closest to him thought he needed strategies beyond those typically provided. Adam learned behaviors more consistent with living an included community lifestyle.

In person-centered planning, support teams start with where a person is, then develop a profile with the person and present it to staff or com-munity members who can help craft a plan that will help to develop a better life for that person. Person-centered planning means helping the person tell about what he or she likes to do and needs and wants in his or her life. Often, it means also exposing the person to different expe-riences because his or her own experiences were so limited.

In 1986, a provider of services to people with disabilities was asked to participate in training on person-centered planning. She was asked to bring along a person who might benefit from such a plan, so she invited Kather-ine. Katherine was 24 years old and had physical challenges from cere-bral palsy in addition to intellectual disabilities. Katherine had been institutionalized since birth, and during her 24 years had lived in a large state-operated institution, in a wing of a nursing home, and now in a facil-ity housing 30 people with severe disabilities. She was quite excited about planning for her future and readily agreed to participate in the planning exercise. Katherine and the service provider talked a lot about Katherine's hopes and dreams: She knew she wanted to live outside of the facility and that she wanted friends and a boyfriend. She smiled and giggled when-ever men came into the facility. The more Katherine and the service provider talked, the more they realized that while Katherine certainly had hopes and dreams, she didn't have enough information to make decisions about them. For example, did she want to live in an apartment or in a house? Did she want to live alone or with others? What kind of work did she want to do? What would be wonderful and special about having a man in her life? Katherine only knew what she had seen on television and what direct support staff had told her about.

As a result of this person-centered, individually focused planning process, Katherine decided that she wanted to first learn more about life in the community. She wanted to go places to meet people, and she wanted to visit different types of apartments and houses and visit with people who actually lived in similar situations so that she could decide what she wanted to do.

The power of the person-centered planning process is that it uncovered what Katherine wanted and gave her a strategy to learn more about how to get it. Instead of the professionals saying what she had to do to get ready, she discovered it for herself.

The Voice of Self-Advocacy

Just as the civil rights movement for racial equality in this country evolved, so did the disability rights movement. People with disabilities and their friends and advocates urged policy makers, professionals, and legislators to develop and fund programs and supports that were based on full inclusion and participation. People with disabilities demanded a seat at their table of planning just as the leaders of the civil rights movements for African Americans took on the leadership of their movement in the 1960s and 1970s. Individuals with disabilities and their families and friends spoke more and more of deciding for themselves what they needed and wanted.

Self Advocates Becoming Empowered (SABE) was created in 1991 when more than 800 self-advocates voted to form a national self-advocacy organization. These individuals, who had been previously "cared for," "done to," and excluded from life, developed a series of principles and goals. Their web site (http://www.sabeusa.org) highlights the following beliefs:

- People with disabilities should be treated as equals.
- People [with disabilities] should be given the same decisions, choices, rights, responsibilities, and chances to speak up and empower themselves.
- People [with disabilities] should be able to make new friendships and renew old friendships just like everyone else.
- People [with disabilities] should be able to learn from their mistakes like everyone else.

SABE's goals include making self-advocacy available in every state to all people with disabilities, including those who live in institutions, go to high schools, reside in rural areas, and live with natural or foster families. SABE also works with people with disabilities about their rights within the criminal justice system. They advocate and are succeeding in closing institutions for people with developmental disabilities nationwide while building community supports.

In September 2005, at the Alliance for Full Participation Summit— a national summit meeting of people involved in the disability field, including self-advocates, family members, policy makers, and professionals—SABE challenged American society to include individuals with disabilities in the full scope of inclusion in society. The agenda for the meeting read, "We belong in schools, neighborhoods, businesses, government and churches, synagogues and mosques. . . . We can all live, work and learn in the community" (Alliance for Full Participation, 2005).

The Role of Direct Support Professionals

Person-centered planning, self-advocacy, and community inclusion are all critical components of the changing focus of the support system for people with disabilities. An additional critical change in the lives of people with disabilities is the role of the direct support professional (DSP). That role evolved much like the rest of the service system. DSPs are the frontline workers and have been called, for example, aides, attendants, caregivers, residential assistants, nursing assistants. Traditionally, their role was to do what they were told by their supervisors. DSPs were assigned to people, shifts, wings, and corridors. Job descriptions included making beds, getting people up and positioned, emptying trash, setting people up with activities, and then moving on. Frontline workers were taught to parrot the words of clinicians about individual goals and objectives when inspectors came to the facility, even though they had little input, information, or understanding about what they were doing, why they were doing it, and most importantly, what it had to do with a person's life.

Today, as people with disabilities move into community life, the reality of having a closely monitored, directly supervised worker is no longer practical, desirable, or possible. Instead, DSPs are the frontline workers who work with a person with disabilities, whether at home, at school, at work, or in community locations. They also work with family members, clinicians, and others who are involved in the life of the person with a disability. DSPs can be caregivers, best friends, advocates, teachers, crisis managers, and facilitators to mention a few of their likely roles.

Because our current person-centered philosophy stresses how important it is to know a person with a disability and what he or she wants, it is logical that the person closest to the person with the disability has a great deal of information to provide about that individual. It is often the DSP—the frontline worker—who receives that information first.

Training of DSPs needed to go beyond first aid, CPR, and the basics of mental retardation and developmental disabilities. In 1996, *The Community Support Skill Standards* were published, redefining the competencies needed by human service workers in contemporary practice (Taylor, Bradley, & Warren, 1996).

The Community Support Skill Standards (CSSS) research project identified the twelve core competencies needed by frontline workers working in the human serviced field. These include:

- Participant empowerment
- Communication

- Assessment
- Community and service networking
- Facilitation of services (planning)
- Community living skills
- Education, training, self development
- Advocacy
- Vocational, educational and career support
- Crisis intervention and prevention
- Organizational participation
- Documentation

These competencies and the skill standards accompanying them are consistent with those needed to help support people with disabilities to reach their fullest capabilities and potential wherever they live and work. These competencies have been the basis for DSP workforce programs around the United States, including the College of Direct Support (see http://www.cds.org) and credentialing programs currently ongoing in many parts of the country (Taylor et al., 1996).

The CSSS competencies are fundamental to the ability of DSPs to support people with disabilities living in the community. DSPs who are with these individuals each day need to help them to make judgments about friendships and relationships, crisis prevention, and safety. DSPs must be trained in a variety of skills and attitudes that will help them understand each individual's wants and needs. An individual with a disability is likely to confide in the DSP about relationships and questions about sexuality, health, and safety.

> As the National Alliance of Direct Support Professionals (NADSP) states in its Code of Ethics, "Direct Support Professionals (DSPs) who support people in their communities are called upon to make independent judgments on a daily basis that involve both practical and ethical reasoning. DSPs have as their mission to follow the individual path suggested by the unique gifts, preferences, and needs of each person they support, and to walk in partnership with the person, and those who love him or her, toward a life of opportunity, well-being, freedom, and contribution." (NADSP, n.d.)

As a result of these significant roles and responsibilities, NADSP's ethical practices include overarching commitments to:

- Person-centered supports
- Promoting physical and emotional well-being
- Integrity and responsibility
- Confidentiality

- Justice, fairness, and equity
- Respect
- Self-determination
- Relationships
- Advocacy

NADSP is also committed to assuring that people have the opportunity to make informed choices in safely expressing their sexuality separating their own personal beliefs and expectations regarding relationships (including sexual relationships) from those desired by other people.

Relationships

Many people with disabilities desire inclusion, to become part of the community, and to have friends, intimacies, and even passion. While it may be very difficult for people with disabilities to develop relationships with others, the consequences of not doing so can be loneliness or the possibility of becoming vulnerable to exploitation.

Agencies that support individuals with disabilities must have policies about inclusion and relationships that are consistent with the law, best practice, individual liberties, and protections. Agencies, schools, and community groups can help individuals with disabilities develop and maintain relationships by providing sex education; anticipating puberty; understanding and, if desirable, preventing reproduction; developing and managing relationships; finding and enjoying reasonable opportunities; and demonstrating assertiveness. Learning how to look nice, go on a date, and act at a party often must be valued and practiced over and over.

Samantha is 29 years old and has Down syndrome. She is the middle child in a supportive, upper-middle class, professional family. When Samantha was 3 years old and her parents were picking a preschool, representatives from the school district suggested a segregated school program. Samantha's parents said, "No. If she is lagging in communication and language, why separate her from typical children?" She was able to attend preschool in a nearby school district. By the time she was 5 years old, Samantha attended the morning kindergarten class and was in a special education class in the afternoon. Her family did not want her to learn sign language, but instead wanted her to learn to speak. To the surprise of many, Samantha learned to read in her kindergarten class.

Fast forward to her life as an adult and see how full it is in work and family and how few outside relationships she has.

Samantha now lives in her own apartment, takes the bus each day to her two jobs, has health insurance, works out, and lives in a convenient, vibrant neighborhood. Her family is struggling to help her develop relationships apart from them. She joined a neighborhood church. Although she tried participating in various social events there, it did not work out well for her. Samantha likes to go to plays at the local theatre, but the bus stops running before the plays are over. The only dance she ever attended was the father/daughter dance at high school.

Samantha is independent, but she is lonely and has not yet experienced her dream for acceptance, companionship, and fun. Samantha's story is unfortunately all too typical.

Mike is 30 years old with severe psychomotor seizures, which are uncontrolled and frequent. He lives in an apartment with two other men and is supported by an agency. While his family is supportive, his parents worry for his safety and his happiness.

Mike and his sister both attended the same high school and were seniors at the same time. His sister and her friends asked if Mike could join them at the prom. His mother was concerned about his seizures, and his sister assured their mother that she and her friends would watch Mike carefully. So, Mike got a tuxedo and joined the group at the prom. He loved it! Mike watched the girls, drank the punch, danced, and was part of the group.

After high school, Mike's sister and her friends went on to college, and Mike continued to live and work in his community. He has no friends, and his mother wonders if he will ever get to a dance again!

In 2004, the Down Syndrome Association of Greater Cincinnati (DSAGC) conducted a major research study to identify, in part, what individuals with Down syndrome and their families considered to be their major unmet needs, in addition to what teachers and social services professionals supporting individuals with Down syndrome considered to be their major unmet needs. The findings of the qualitative (e.g., focus groups) and quantitative (e.g., surveys) research performed by DSAGC further demonstrate the importance of relationships to people with Down syndrome and their families.

In the focus groups, adults with Down syndrome reported that they wanted to be considered typical people, wanted to be in the community, wanted marriage, and wanted good jobs. Many reported that "a lack of communication skills" and the "fear of being disliked" interfered with their aspirations to be out in the community leading typical lives. They reported that they felt well-liked, but had gained that acceptance through being overly agreeable and compliant and by not "rocking the boat." They also reported that they had few friends outside of their families, and even fewer romantic involvements, and they had no one to confide in. Statements such as "I keep to myself" and "I talk to my rosary" communicate the isolation they experienced daily. Most of the participants reported that their leisure time was spent alone even though they wanted interaction and connection with both typical adults and adults with disabilities (Rugen, 2004).

Parents of both adults and children with Down syndrome reported similar frustrations at helping their children connect and develop more inclusive relationships in the community. While there are many wonderful stories of inclusion and involvement, there are still major gaps in including people with disabilities in all aspects of life. Parents of children with Down syndrome report stories of their child's exclusion and isolation from others. As one parent revealed, "Kids don't want to play with my son because he is rough. He doesn't know how to interact." Their efforts to develop play dates with typically developing children were reported to be unsuccessful and resulted in further hurt and rejection for their children. Similarly, teachers of young children with Down syndrome reported rejection and isolation of their students, even in inclusive classes (Rugen, 2004).

This research clearly points to a gap between the expectation of inclusion and acceptance and the reality experienced by participants in DSAGC's 2004 research study. Attitudes of families and friends impact this dynamic even further and can result in happier more fulfilling outcomes.

Jason, a 43-year-old man with a mild intellectual disability and behavioral challenges, and Sara, a 40-year-old woman with Down syndrome, had been a couple for years; however, marriage always seemed far off and unworkable. When holidays came around, Jason visited his family and Sara visited her family. The sex educator that worked with the organization that provided supports to this couple suggested that they start acting more like a typical couple so that their families could see them and support them in their relationship. So, like millions of couples and families everywhere, they began to alternate holidays between their families. Their families experienced them as a couple and saw their maturity and love and how their relationship added to both their individual and family lives. It worked, and Jason and Sara eventually got married.

Implications of Community Inclusion and Self-Determination

Now that more people with disabilities are included in the mainstream of society and given the opportunity to make their own choices and decisions and freely participate in the community, they and those closest to them are faced with the benefits and consequences of their actions. The benefits and risks inherent in living in the community affect people with disabilities, but they cannot be considered a barrier to their freedom to live in communities of their choosing.

Now that institutionalization is not a common option, the challenge for people with disabilities and those who help support them is to balance the risks, responsibilities, and freedom against cognitive and physical realties that may interfere with leading a full life. Risks include those inherent in an active life in the community including exploitation, sexually transmitted diseases, consent, safety, and civil rights. This is no small task!

Michael Smull, a leader in the development, expansion, and refinement of person-centered planning, cautions us to balance what is important *to* with what is important *for* the person with an intellectual or developmental disability (Smull, 2003). A balance between health and safety and choice and responsibility must be found. The more we get to know people, the more likely we are to help them achieve that balance in life. With sexuality, the consequences of losing that balance can be quite serious.

We know that the world can be a rather unsafe place. In the 1970s, we thought that most of the physical risks of increased sexuality could be addressed through birth control and the right to an abortion. Of course, this was to be coupled with sex education, moral and ethical responsibility, and good decision making on the part of each individual and his or her friends and advocates. We know, however, that this does not always happen. Richard Sobsey's research on violence and abuse for people with disabilities revealed that, as society began to speak more freely about sex, we learned that sexual abuse was much more frequently occurring than had been expected, and was much more frequently occurring among people with developmental disabilities than among their peers without disabilities, in both their own homes and in residential facilities. The consequences of both consensual and nonconsensual sexual relationships were increased with the new risks identified including unintended pregnancies and HIV/AIDS, herpes, and other sexually transmitted diseases.

As people with disabilities are finally being given the opportunity to make their own choices and decisions through person-centered planning and changes in attitudes, these rights must be balanced against the very serious risks of these activities. Decisions that result in increased vulnerability and/or those that result from choices made by vulnerable, lonely people looking for love and relationships can have consequences that can influence the whole trajectory of their life. Many people with intellectual disabilities supported through the service system do require support to make decisions. Individuals with disabilities, their families, friends, DSPs, and advocates must become familiar with laws of consent and the long- and short-term implications of the choices they make. Person-centered planning and inclusion for people with disabilities is not meant to expose people to risks and situations for which they have not been prepared.

Every state in the country has laws governing a person's ability to make decisions about sexuality. The goals of the laws are to protect people from harm, rather than limit their opportunities. (A more in-depth discussion on consent is presented in Chapter 9.) This balance of facilitating choice and inclusion will require ongoing vigilance and attention to support people with disabilities to lead the lives they choose. This is not the same as readiness discussed earlier—it is not saying that a person must achieve a certain skill or cognitive level to experience relationships—however, it is critically important that an individual with disabilities learn how to make suitable judgments in sit-uations and that their support system be designed to promote both opportunity and safety.

As people with disabilities develop intimate relationships, for example, the issues of birth control, parenting, and raising children emerge. These issues have not been resolved and involve deeply per-sonal, religious, ethical, and practical considerations. In previous gen-erations, when intimate unions of people with disabilities produced children, these children were automatically removed from their house-hold to be raised by others. We know today that planning and educa-tion and supports can make a difference in that outcome. Now that states are no longer able to just say "We're taking the baby," the issues remain complex:

- Does the individual with a disability want the child?

- Are prospective parents with disabilities taught about the different options available (e.g., abortion, raising the child, supports needed and available, adoption by a family member, adoption by an out-sider)?

- Can the parent care for a child?

- Are supports available to assure health, safety, and nurturing for the child?

- What happens when the child's cognitive abilities surpass those of his or her parents?

- What happens if there is a complex disability that is passed geneti-cally to the child?

A deep respect for individuals with disabilities to make their own informed choices and experience the same rights as people in the community at large must be balanced with the reality of the difficulty of raising a child, emotionally, financially, and intellectually. Certainly, people with disabilities who wish to raise and nurture children should receive needed supports to help them do so. Recent movies, such as *I Am Sam* and *The Other Sister*, have addressed some of these issues. The following chapter in this book presents in-depth stories about relationships told by couples with disabilities and will provide more insight from their points of view.

CONCLUSION

This last story about Zelda provides a snapshot of the challenges and dilemmas that people with disabilities and their friends and support people face as they move into the community and have the freedom of developing their own friendships and relationships. Think about the many conflicting and critical issues raised as you think about Zelda's choices and decisions and the responsibilities and ethical challenges faced by those closest to her in her life.

Zelda is 30 years old and has mild intellectual disabilities. Zelda has her own apartment and rides the bus to and from work; Zelda is very independent and successful. In addition to her full-time job, Zelda is involved in a romantic relationship with a man in another city. Zelda has a strong network of support both in her community and from her family who nervously allow Zelda to live far from them.

In the past, Zelda has made some poor judgments about people who come into her life, especially men. These poor judgments resulted in actions that caused emotional setbacks and potential dangers for Zelda.

For example, a man she did not know well invited her over one evening. They were talking, and the man offered to give her a massage. She readily agreed, and Zelda enjoyed this interaction several times, initially with her blouse on and later with her blouse off. She reciprocated by giving the man massages as well.

After a few more evenings the man told Zelda that men enjoyed having their penises touched. He asked if she had ever heard the word "semen." Zelda said she had never heard that word before. He told her that men liked to have their penises massaged and sucked until semen was released.

When Zelda told her older friends and mentors about these events, they told her that she should not go to the man's apartment again. Her friend, Angela, reminded Zelda that she was in a serious relationship already and reviewed many of the things that Zelda had learned about sex and relationships. Angela talked of love and safety and responsibility. Zelda agreed not to see the man again.

But that advice made Zelda unhappy and reminded her that she would be lonely without the man's company and massages. Zelda spoke with her counselor and support provider. They both told her that she was her own guardian and she should do what she liked. They told Zelda that if she wanted to participate in those activities, she could see the man again. It was her choice. Zelda liked that answer better and told Angela what the others had said. Angela did try to report the incident, but since Zelda was older than 21 and is her own guardian, there was no legal way to prevent Zelda from making the choice to see the man.

Zelda recounted this incident to several different people in her circle of support and received contradictory advice from each of them!

How can Zelda figure out what is the right balance between safety and personal freedom? How can the people who care about Zelda balance safety and personal freedom? Is Zelda using sexual activity that may be exploitive or even dangerous to meet a need that could be better met another way? Is legal intervention the only recourse in supporting Zelda? What is Zelda communicating about her life?

As we have seen in this brief discussion, the change in the service structure and philosophy of services has caused a major shift in thinking about people with disabilities. More and more, people with intellectual disabilities live in the community and are exposed to the same opportunities and challenges as the rest of society. Human sexuality, relationships, intimacy, funding, and rights and responsibilities must be considered as people plan for their lives. With thousands more people with disabilities living in the community than in the past, and with thousands more on the waiting list for services and supports, society as a whole, professionals, clinicians, advocates, and self-advocates will be faced with difficult decisions and choices. Initiatives such as those of The Arc of Minnesota "to unlock the waiting list" have increased the number of people living in sites funded by the Home and Community Based Waiver in Minnesota from 7,607 in 2000 to 14,514 in 2002 (Braddock et al., 2004). The corresponding financial and societal impact for these people as well as the thousands of others on waiting lists across the country will require difficult choices in the years to come. It is important that policy and personal decisions be made with a full understanding of how the system has changed and evolved over the past 40 years. The issues presented in this book related to personal choice, responsibility, implications of intimacy, sexuality, and relationships are critical and must remain in the forefront as planning is done in the future.

REFERENCES

Alliance for Full Participation. (2005). *Agenda for full participation in America.* Available at: http://www.thearc.org/AFPAgenda.pdf

Braddock, D., Hemp, R., & Rizzolo, M.C. (2004, October). State of the States in developmental disabilities: 2004. *Mental Retardation, 42*(5), 356–370.

Burton, B. & Kaplan, F. (1974). *Christmas in purgatory: A photographic essay on mental retardation.* Syracuse, NY: Syracuse University, Center on Human Policy.

Education for All Handicapped Children Act of 1975, PL 94-142, 20 U.S.C. §§ 1400 *et seq.*

Duggar, C. (1993, March 12). Big day for ex-residents of the Center for the Retarded. *The New York Times,* pp. A1, A3.

Hewitt, A., O'Nell, S. (1998). Speaking up–speaking out. President's Committee on Mental Retardation. In Y. Bestgen (Ed.), *With a little help from my friends: A series on contemporary supports to people with mental retardation.* Towson, MD: National Committee on Outcomes Resources. Retrieved August 29, 2006, from http://www.ncor.org/AuthorsBk1.html

Individuals with Disabilities Education Act of 1990, PL 101-476, 20 U.S.C. §§ 1400 *et seq.*

O'Brien, J., & O'Brien, C.L. (1992). *Contrasting approaches.* Policy Bulletin #3. Syracuse, New York: Center on Human Policy.

Rehabilitation Act of 1973, PL 93-112, 29 U.S.C. §§ 701 *et seq.*

Rugen, B. (2004). *Report on strategic focus group research.* Cincinnati, OH: Down Syndrome Association of Greater Cincinnati.

Schlesinger, A.M. (1978). *Robert Kennedy and his times.* Boston: Houghton Mifflin.

Sobsey, R. (1999). *Educational psychology.* Baltimore: Paul H. Brookes Publishing Co.

Smull, M. (2003). Helping people be happy and safe: Accounting for health and safety in how people want to live. In V.J. Bradley & D.S.W. Kimmich (Eds.), *Quality enhancement in developmental disabilities: Challenges and opportunities in a changing world* (pp. 121–160). Baltimore: Paul H. Brookes Publishing Co.

State Operations Manual Department of Health and Human Services Code of Federal Regulations, 483.440

National Alliance of Direct Support Professionals Code of Ethics. Retrieved August 29, 2006, from http://www.nadsp.org/library/codetext.asp

Taub, S.L., Smith, G.A., & Bradley, V.J. (2003). The national core indicators project: Monitoring the performance of state developmental disabilities agencies. In V.J. Bradley & D.S.W. Kimmich (Eds.), *Quality enhancement in developmental disabilities: Challenges and opportunities in a changing world.* Baltimore: Paul H. Brookes Publishing Co.

Taylor, M., Bradley, V., & Warren, R. (1996). *The community support skill standards: Tools for managing change and achieving outcomes.* Cambridge, MA: Human Services Research Institute.

6

In Their Own Words

Couples Tell Their Stories

Nancy Parello(with photographs by Shay Platz)

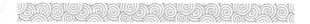

It was a sticky summer day, the kind made for swimming in a backyard pool. Jerome had left behind the darkness of the institution where he spent his childhood and far too many years of his adult life. On this day, though, he had no worries of being tied to his bed or of being beaten by the other boys at the hospital.

He was in a real backyard, with a deck, a pool, a dog, and a friend. He ran along the deck, feeling its slippery wetness beneath his bare feet, the pool shimmering beside him. It was a perfect day, full of promise, hope and, most of all, escape. Then the ground slipped out from beneath him. He hit hard against the deck and bounced into the cold pool. Jerome started to sink, the clear, chlorinated water swallowing him.

The young girl, Lorraine, called to her mother for help. But the sight of her friend slipping below the surface terrified her so much that she forgot about herself. She jumped into the water, her German shepherd, Lady, splashing in behind her.

"Me and Lady, we saved him," Lorraine says.

Now, many years later, Jerome and Lorraine are engaged. And they are, in a sense, still saving each other. Jerome has learned how to call 911 and what to say if Lorraine has a seizure. Lorraine is teaching Jerome how to read.

Special thanks and recognition to the administration and members of Community Access Unlimited of New Jersey for their generosity in sharing their stories.

Their history, their hopes, and their needs bind them together, in many ways, like any couple. But, for them, the simple fact that they live together in a smart apartment in a northeastern suburban town, where Lorraine's wedding dress waits in the closet, is beyond anything either could have imagined. So far are they from the shadows of institutions, boarding houses, and foster homes. And, the stigma of having intellectual disabilities.

Now Jerome and Lorraine have a freedom and a normalcy that leaves them coping with many of the same issues any other couple faces. Who's going to clean the kitchen? Sweep the floor? Do the laundry? What will we have for dinner? How should we spend the holidays?

As people with intellectual disabilities increasingly find their place in the world, they are also entering relationships and learning to deal with the joy and the pain of loving another human being. To learn more about how the theories of relationships play out in the messy reality of life, we interviewed several couples to gain a deeper understanding of their relationships, their lives, their struggles, and their dreams.

Here are their stories, as they told them to me.

JEROME AND LORRAINE

Jerome and Lorraine met as children, living in separate large institutions that shared social dances once each month.

Jerome, now 44, never knew his parents or any members of his family. He spent his early years in foster homes. In his preadolescent years, he began having behavioral troubles. When he was 13, he was sent to a now-defunct institution. He was later moved to another facility, this one at the other end of the state.

Lorraine, now 50, was luckier. She spent her childhood in a suburban home in the central part of the same state as Jerome. She was protected by her mother and was part of a large family. But, when Lorraine became a teenager, the task of caring for her became too much for her mother to handle. Her mother finally decided to place her in an institution, not far from where Jerome was living.

"She didn't put me away because she didn't love me," Lorraine explains. "She'd visit every 2 weeks."

Sometimes, Lorraine's mother would take her home for visits, and Lorraine would ask if Jerome could come along. They brought him home to celebrate the holidays, and Lorraine's family included him in family picnics. It was Jerome's only memories of having a real home, with people who cared about him.

"Everybody liked Jerome," Lorraine remembers.

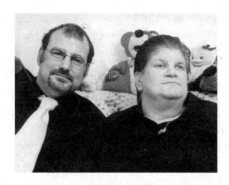

Over the years, the two float-ed in and out of each other's lives, as they moved from home to home. When Lorraine left her institutional placement, she stayed in boarding houses and foster homes for a while. It was at one of these places that Lorraine first experienced sex. The son of the woman who ran the home raped her.

The rape resulted in a pregnancy. When Lorraine was 34, she gave birth to a baby boy. "I couldn't think of a name, so my foster mother named him."

The state's child protection agency took Lorraine's son from her when he was 4 1/2 years old. At that point, the boy was living with Lor-raine's foster mother, while Lorraine was living with her brother. One day, she tried to call her foster mother and discovered that the phone number was disconnected. She has not seen her son since, although she has searched for him for years. He is now 16, and Lorraine fervently hopes to find him before she and Jerome get married so that he can attend the ceremony.

Even though Lorraine was unable to care for her son, she loved him and tried, as best she could, to provide for him. She gave $100 to her fos-ter mother to put in his savings account. "I want him to go to college," Lorraine says.

No one—not Lorraine's mother, teachers, or friends—ever talked to her about sex, so she had no idea what to expect or what to do. She also knew nothing about birth control or protecting herself from sexu-ally transmitted infections. And, even though her first sexual encounter was forced, she shrugs it off, almost as though it is supposed to be that way. She expresses no anger or pain over the rape incident.

"He woke me up at 5 in the morning," she remembers, matter-of-factly. "I didn't feel a thing. I was asleep."

After she lost her son, Lorraine lived with one of her brothers in a seaside town in the same state. There, she learned about how hurtful love could be. Her brother managed a motel and Lorraine would clean the rooms. She got involved with one of her brother's friends, who would also help with the cleaning.

Their relationship was tumultuous. They fought often. He hit her on several occasions. The last time, he threw her against the wall. Lor-raine finally phoned another brother, who called the police.

"He used to beat the hell out of me all the time," Lorraine remem-bers. "He used to go out with so many girls, beating the hell out of them."

After that, Lorraine steered clear of men for a long time—until she and Jerome found each other again, both now in programs run by a nonprofit agency in their state that helps people with mental and/or intellectual disabilities integrate into the community and exercise self-determination.

Jerome was happy to meet up with Lorraine again. After spending most of his life in institutions, he was finally liberated in 1993. This very same agency helped him find an apartment and a job. With supports to navigate the outside world, Jerome is evidence of the ability of a person with a significant intellectual disability to live a full life outside of institutional walls.

Jerome dated a couple of girls during the many years he lived in an institution. He had his first girlfriend when he was a teenager. They got along at first, but, like many adolescent relationships, they began to argue. Jerome's girlfriend did not like the fact that he smoked. And she was jealous of other girls. "She didn't want me to go with nobody else," Jerome remembers.

He had his first sexual encounter with a girl named Paula. They were friends. And Paula took the lead. Jerome remembers the experience as being friendly, comfortable. Even though he took a sex education course at the institution and he learned about using condoms, Jerome said he has not used them every time he has sex. He often does not have any on hand. Plus, Jerome says he prefers sex without condoms.

Jerome, like Lorraine, never had a truly committed relationship before the two of them got together back in 1999. They met again at a social gathering, organized by the agency that provided support to them. Lorraine was feeling ill that night, and Jerome noticed. He asked for her phone number. The next morning, he called to check on his old friend.

"He called early Saturday morning," Lorraine remembers. "I said, 'Why are you calling me this early? What the hell did you wake me up for?'"

"I was calling to see if you're feeling better," Jerome says now.

And so, they once again began looking out for each other. The two childhood friends became reacquainted. They continued their friendship. At some point—neither could say exactly when—the friendship grew into something more. They had their first "real date" on New Year's Eve.

"I paid for her," Jerome remembers. "She had no money."

"My brother don't give me that much money," Lorraine explains.

"We've been friends for a while," Jerome says. "Then we changed to boyfriend and girlfriend. Me and Lorraine talked. We didn't rush into it. We got to be patient with each other."

"You got to get to know each other," Lorraine adds.

"You need to know what each other likes," Jerome agrees. "You got to know what she likes."

Pretty soon, the relationship turned physical. They had sex for the first time in the apartment that Jerome then shared with two roommates. Lorraine remembers feeling relaxed and comfortable with Jerome. Since they had known each other for so long, neither felt embarrassed. Lorraine's only worry was that Jerome's roommates might walk in on them.

"I told Jerome to lock the door," she remembers.

They did not use protection—condoms or any other type of birth control—even though both say they knew they should. Lorraine figured she was too old to get pregnant, she says. And Jerome said he still preferred sex without condoms.

The couple dated for many years, spending nights at each other's apartment. It was a hassle, Jerome remembers. "I'd have to go back and forth and bring my stuff—vitamins, medications," he says. "Now I see her all the time. I like being able to be together all the time."

It took some doing to get the couple under the same roof. They were in different programs and, because they were not married, they depended on their agency to overcome these obstacles. They needed agency staff to advocate for them to achieve their dream of living together.

Now, they are planning to be married. They hesitate because if they marry, Lorraine risks decreasing her Social Security. This is the marriage penalty in action. So they are probably going to have a commitment ceremony in June. They have been busy planning the affair, which will be held in a place that is large enough for their friends and family members to all attend and wish them well.

Lorraine sips coffee from a mug, with a Santa Claus on it, sitting in her comfortable kitchen, with new cabinets and appliances and a picture of her and Jerome hanging on the refrigerator. She puffs a cigarette, wearing a yellow, hooded sweatshirt. And she talks about their life together and the wedding they are planning.

Like a couple who has been married for years, they quarrel, but with a familiarity that says they know these little disagreements are nothing compared to the commitment they feel for each other. Lorraine chides Jerome for failing to tend to his chores around the apartment. Jerome tells Lorraine to stop interrupting when he is trying to tell a story.

But both say they rarely have heated arguments. When things get tense, Lorraine tells Jerome to go outside and have a cigarette. He does. And then when he comes back, they work through their differences, both say.

Jerome and Lorraine seem to understand that, far more important than the little quarrels, is the fact that their relationship is grounded in the help and support they give each other every day, each wanting to fill the other's needs, large and small.

Jerome goes into his room and produces a computer that Lorraine bought him for Christmas. They are using technology to teach Jerome how to read. Lorraine is also showing Jerome how to figure out the train schedules so that he can get around more easily. And, she is helping him learn how to manage money, figuring out a monthly budget. The two share the bills, with Jerome paying the cable bill and Lorraine paying the phone bill. They both buy food. Their agency finances the rent.

Jerome, in turn, has learned how to call 911 and what information he must give to help Lorraine, in the event that she has a seizure, a worry that had weighed heavily upon Lorraine before she had Jerome next to her. "Lorraine would ask, 'What happens if I have a seizure? Who's going to call 911?"

The two are busy planning their wedding.

Jerome produces a small white box and carefully lifts its lid. Inside, snug against the blue velvet, is a ring, thin, etched gold, with a small diamond in the middle. It's beautiful. Lorraine smiles.

"I bought this for her for Christmas," Jerome says.

"I paid for it," Lorraine returns.

"No you didn't," he answers.

"I'm saving to buy him a wedding band," Lorraine says, ending the argument.

Lorraine gets up from the kitchen table and walks into her neat bedroom, which is separate from Jerome's. Stuffed animals sit in a row along the headboard of her bed. She opens the double-door closet and carefully takes out a dress, wrapped in plastic. She lovingly lifts the plastic to reveal a white wedding dress, with a band of pearls around the bodice. Jerome stands at the bedroom door and watches.

They look at each other, but neither speaks. No words of love. No displays of affection. But you know that together, the two of them will find their way, for all the days of their lives.

NATALIE AND RALPH

The apartment is cluttered, boxes still unpacked from the recent move, clothes strewn on the couch. The little boy lies on the dirty carpet. His mother kneels next to him, lifts his bare behind and tries to wipe the toddler. But the boy lashes out and scratches his mother's arm. She snaps up and raises her hand as if to slap the child in the face, but she stops herself. The child starts to howl.

The father stands over the two of them and chides his wife for losing her temper with the child. Then, he leans over and reprimands the child who is too young to understand the words. The boy cries even harder. He must have understood the tone of his father's voice and recognized the impatience of his parents. We all wait tensely while the mother struggles to secure a new diaper on her crying child.

Evan is 2 years old, and by far, the greatest challenge—and the greatest gift—of Natalie and Ralph's marriage. While the couple had talked about having children, they never really got to the point where they made a decision. Like many couples, it just happened. They were both surprised.

"With all the women I'd been with, I didn't think I was fertile," Ralph says, explaining why they never used birth control.

When Ralph, 34, and Natalie, 33, found out they were pregnant, they knew the risks were considerable. Natalie has suffered from grand mal seizures ever since she was a child. While the medication she takes helps control the seizures, it could have caused serious birth defects to her unborn child.

"The doctors told us that he could be born with a hole in his heart, a hole in his spine, or muscular dystrophy," Natalie says. "That was my biggest challenge. Living with the fear that he might not be healthy or he might not survive. I was scared."

"But we did not want to abort this baby," Ralph said.

"I said, no, I'm not stopping it," adds Natalie, "I'm taking my chances. And he came out fine. He's a little slow with speech and walking. Other than that, he's fine."

Since it was a high-risk birth, a specialist monitored Natalie's entire pregnancy. Starting in her second trimester, she had a blood test every month to test the baby's health. Ralph went with Natalie to every prenatal appointment, holding his wife's hand, providing constant support. He marvels now at her fortitude.

"The pregnancy never slowed this woman down," he says.

"Toward the end, I was walking slow," she corrects him.

They were together in the delivery room. Natalie was able to have a vaginal delivery. And Ralph was the first person in the world to hold their little boy. "That was the best part," he says.

When Natalie and baby Evan came home from the hospital, Ralph took off from work so that he could care for his son and wife for the first week or so. "I was taking care of two invalids," he remembers. "The first night, I cooked. I set off the smoke alarms. The place was filled with smoke, and I thought, 'There go the pork chops.'"

Natalie took it in stride. "She said, 'Order pizza!'" Ralph remembers.

Like most new parents, they had to learn how to care for their infant. They learned how to diaper the boy. "I learned to keep the diaper over his penis when you're changing him so you don't get squirt," Ralph says.

Fortunately for all, they had some help. A friend of the family stayed with them in the first few months, teaching them how to care for an infant and helping them learn to cope with the challenges of parenting. It has been a difficult journey, complicated by the couple's disabilities, they said.

"Because of our disabilities, being a child myself, it's hard for me to be the heavy, to put rules down," Ralph says. "There are times when I'm frustrated. Evan is frustrated. My wife gets cranky. We'll have a fight. Sometimes my temper can get the best of me. But she knows I love her."

Natalie says she tries to avoid confrontation. "I just go in my room," she says.

"Oh, please, you can fight with the best of them, lady," Ralph challenges. Natalie just shrugs.

Money is tight. They didn't realize how expensive a little child could be. They have had a lot of help. Their support agency purchased a number of items for the baby, including a crib. State workers brought a monitor, a case of formula, and a box of diapers. The couple gets child care assistance from the state, but they may soon face a co-pay, as their income has risen. They pay $138 a month in rent, and utilities run about $100 a month. They both work and receive some other government assistance.

Natalie's mother helps out, too. But, shortly after Evan was born, Ralph was laid off because he missed a lot of work, staying home to help his wife with the baby. Their agency again came to the rescue, providing Ralph with a janitorial job, cleaning members' houses.

"I love working for this agency, as well as being a member," he says, clearly appreciative.

Both Ralph and Natalie spent their early years at home with their respective families. Ralph got in trouble when he was a teenager and spent some time in juvenile detention. "My parents disowned me," he says. He hasn't seen his parents since he was 17. But Natalie's mother lives close by and is very involved with the couple and with her grandson.

When Natalie first met Ralph at a mutual friend's house, she was wary. He was always kidding around, joking with her. She was more seri-

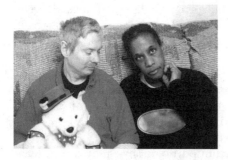

ous. And she didn't know if she could trust him. It took a little convincing, but Natalie finally agreed to go out with Ralph. They quickly realized that each had something to offer the other.

"She knew more things than I did," Ralph said. "She was the kind of person I wanted to know. I knew I was never going to find anyone better than Natalie. She was more mature in the way she carried herself. It leveled me out. It complemented my comedy side. I knew she was right for me."

"I like the way he treats me, and how he doesn't take everything seriously," Natalie says.

They had their first date in October 1999 at a gala awards dinner/dance, attended by local politicians. They were engaged two months later, on New Year's Eve. They moved in together shortly after they became engaged. The agency went to great pains and worked it out so that Natalie could live in Ralph's apartment, with him and his two roommates. They moved into their own apartment shortly before they were married in August 2000.

In their short marriage, the two came dangerously close to tragedy.

It was Super Bowl Sunday in 2001, just 5 months after they had married. Natalie wasn't feeling well. She and Ralph had cleaned up the apartment. They were expecting company to come over and watch the game with them. Ralph went into the bedroom to take a short nap before their guests arrived. When he awoke and went out into the living room, Natalie was lying on the floor.

"I knew about the seizures, but I didn't know the symptoms," he explains.

Ralph helped her to the couch and went to call for help. While he was dialing the phone, he heard a crash from the living room. He raced in to find Natalie on the floor, the coffee table overturned. Natalie was having another seizure. He was terrified.

"I thought I was going to be a widower," Ralph says.

"I was this close to dying," Natalie adds.

Ralph dialed 911. Luckily, the hospital was located just blocks away. The EMTs arrived quickly. Natalie was unconscious in the ambulance. Ralph sat beside her, holding her hand, praying. When they arrived at the hospital, Natalie awoke and started screaming. As the medical team was wheeling her to get a CAT scan, she began having another seizure.

The doctors finally were able to stabilize her. Natalie spent nearly 1 week in the hospital, while Ralph stayed by her side, helping to nurse her back to health. It is a fear he lives with now every day.

"I fear for her because, yes, she can have a grand mal seizure again," Ralph says.

Both Ralph and Natalie say that they had no formal sexuality training. Ralph's mother told him about the mechanics of sex, but she used insults to try to keep him from having it. "She just said, 'Don't do it. We don't want any more dumb kids running around.'"

So, Ralph learned about sex from pornography—movies and magazines—and books. Natalie's mother also discouraged her from having sex. "She just told me not to do it." Of course, neither listened.

Ralph's first sexual encounter came on a cruise ship when he was 21. A friend fixed him up with a woman, who made him use condoms. He was tense the first time, unsure of what to do and afraid he would be unable to please his partner. "I felt like I needed to loosen up," he says. "I was shy about it. I felt funny the first time. I didn't know if I was hurting her. But I was curious. The woman took her time with me. She showed me how to make her happy. She taught me everything I needed to know."

They continued a relationship for about 2 months after the cruise was over, but gradually separated, parting friends.

Natalie was 18 when she had sex for the first time with a boyfriend who was 2 years younger. She had been dating the boy for about 2 months when he began pressuring her to have sex. She was unsure whether she really wanted to take that step, but she was also afraid to say no.

"He wanted to get an adult movie," she remembers. "He was too young, so he asked me if I would get it. I got the movie."

They went to the basement of his parents' house and, while his parents were at work, they watched the movie and had sex on the couch. Natalie was scared. "I didn't know what it would be like," she says. "It was OK. It wasn't that great. He probably didn't know what he was doing."

While her first experience was unplanned and unprotected, she says she has no real regrets. But, she also says that later experiences were more satisfying. "Other boyfriends did it a lot better," she says.

When she and Ralph first started dating, they decided to wait a little while before having sex. "I respect that she didn't want to have sex right away. I understood that," Ralph said.

The first time they had sex, they were at Natalie's mother's house, while she was out dancing. They didn't really discuss it beforehand. "We just thought our relationship was strong enough," says Ralph. Ralph was afraid Natalie's mother would walk in. Natalie says she felt "really comfortable" with Ralph, more comfortable than with anyone else she had ever been with.

"It was better than with the other girls," Ralph adds. "Natalie handled the sexual part better. She let me take my time."

Now, with the demands of raising a child, the two say their sex life has ground to a near halt. Neither could remember the last time that they made love. "Let's just say Evan eats up all our energy," Ralph says.

When they do have sex, though, they often forego the birth control. Although Ralph says he's a "firm believer" in birth control, he also says they just don't always get around to buying it. Most of the time, he withdraws. But, both say they might be ready to have another baby, anyway.

"If God blesses us with another healthy baby boy, then we'll take that," Ralph says. "If we get a baby with a birth defect, then we'll deal with that, too."

CHARLES AND GEORGINA

Charles calls her GG and tries to convince her to marry him. He wants them to live together, in their own apartment, where they can make the rules. She shrugs her shoulders and says, "I'm not the type to get married."

But Charles won't let it go that easily.

"We can make it," he assures her.

She shakes her head and stares at her hands, resting on the kitchen table. "We gotta learn a lot of things if we get married," Georgina says.

Charles lets it go—for now. After all, the two have a happy relationship, sharing a kind of quiet companionship that serves them well at this stage of their lives. Charles, 70, and Georgina, 64, live two floors away from each other in a supervised apartment program. They each have a nice, newly renovated two-bedroom apartment. Georgina shares her apartment with Debbie. Charles lives with John.

The couple spends most evenings together, watching television, sometimes sharing dinner and helping each other with chores. Charles often helps Georgina carry the groceries up the three flights of steps to her apartment. On the weekends, they occasionally go out to lunch. Sometimes, they take walks around the neighborhood or go to the local pizza parlor. Other times, Georgina's sister comes and treats the couple to dinner.

Charles goes to church on Sundays. Georgina spends her days working at an occupational center. Charles is still hoping to find a job because he gets bored during the day, waiting for Georgina to return.

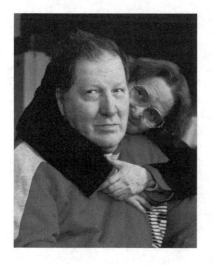

They rarely argue, but when they do, it passes quickly.

"One time he told me to get out of here," Georgina remembers. "I left until it passed."

"We get along good," adds Charles, his blue eyes resting warmly on the woman he clearly loves. "We've been together for a long time."

Charles's biggest complaint is Georgina's roommate. The two often get into arguments, so Charles tries to avoid going upstairs to Georgina's apartment. He also bemoans the fact that they have to abide by the curfews that are a condition of living in the supervised apartment program. The rules say residents must be in their own apartments by 9 P.M.

But, Charles has convinced the staff to allow him and Georgina an extra hour together at night. Still, many nights, Charles wants to stay with Georgina. "It would be nice if we had our own apartment," he says. She, however, is quite content with their arrangement and so she gently rebuffs his attempts to change their living situation. "No, no, no," she mumbles, her words barely audible.

Neither Charles nor Georgina had much experience in relationships prior to meeting each other years ago through the supervised apartment program. Georgina lived at home with her mother for her entire life. She was relatively shielded from many outside influences and had little opportunity to meet men. She did have one boyfriend, many years ago, when she attended a school in another city. "Mom never talked about men," Georgina says.

When Georgina's mother died, her sister scouted for a community program and placed Georgina in the apartment where she lives now.

Charles spent his early adult years living in an institution. He doesn't like to talk about it. He shuts his eyes tight, and shakes his head, the pain of the memory showing in his deeply lined face. "It was no good," he says simply. "It feels good to be in your own apartment and be on your own."

Charles also had one other girlfriend, a woman he met while living in a different supervised apartment program. "I didn't like her," he says now. "She came after me."

Neither Charles nor Georgina ever had any children.

"I can't take care of myself," Georgina says. "It's hard to take care of kids. I wouldn't know what to do."

Sex is also something they have decided to forego, its complications too much for either of them to even contemplate. Instead, they live a quiet, simple life together, comfortable in the knowledge that they have a familiar hand to hold, as they grow old together.

SHERRY AND AL

Sherry was alone in the apartment on that cold winter day when the telephone rang and Al's brother relayed the bad news. The father of her live-in boyfriend Al had died. Sherry knew that Al and his father were very close. She realized the news would devastate him.

Al was at the mall, playing video games, one of his favorite pastimes. Sherry wasn't sure when he would be home. But she knew that he should hear the news from his family. So she bundled up in her warm parka and headed to the bus stop to wait for Al to come home. When he finally stepped off the bus, he was a little curious that she was waiting for him. But Sherry just told him that she wanted to take him to a friend of the family, who lived close by. They walked there together. When Al heard the news, he broke down.

"He wasn't good," Sherry remembers. "He was crying hysterically. I hugged him, but that didn't stop him from crying."

Al remembers feeling comforted, though, that Sherry was with him. "It made me happy," he says.

The two have been a couple for 12 years. They both love the Yankees. They argue over whether they argue. (Al says they don't argue. Sherry says they do.) They tried living together once, but it didn't work out. Still, they can't imagine life without the other.

"I love Al very much," Sherry says simply. "I don't ever want to lose Al."

"Aw, honeybear," Al returns.

The two first met at a social function sponsored by the community-based agency where they were both clients. A mutual friend introduced them. It was her feet that first attracted Al to his sweetheart Sherry. "He calls my feet 'babies,'" Sherry says. For Sherry, it was Al's easy, friendly manner that made her take a shine to her honey. Even so, their first date was a disaster. It was so bad that neither wants to talk about what happened. But, something drew them back to each other, to try again—and has kept them together for the past 12 years.

They have similar backgrounds. Both spent most of their childhood living with a loving, protective family. Each went away to school for several years during adolescence. And both have been living in the community for years, largely managing their own lives, working, and making friends. So, after their initial dating disaster, their friendship quickly turned into a more intimate relationship. After several years, Al and Sherry tired of traveling back and forth between each other's apartments. They decided they wanted to live together.

But, they had two hurdles to overcome before they could rest their heads on the same pillow each night. Namely, their mothers. Both Al's and Sherry's moms were wary of the two sharing an apartment, fearing that they were not up to handling the demands of such a full-time relationship. But, Al and Sherry were persistent. They finally convinced the concerned mothers that they could handle it. The mothers imposed one condition, though. Al had to get a vasectomy. He is still bitter about being forced to make such a personal decision.

"My mother said I had to do it if I wanted to live with Sherry," he says. "I was mad at her. I wanted to have a family. I still do. But they didn't think we could handle it."

"I think we could," Sherry says. "It's a lot of responsibility. I would need help."

"We could do it, honey," Al says, with the eagerness of a child.

Both complain that their mothers interfere too much in their relationship. They feel as if they are treated like children instead of adults. And they wish they were allowed to have more control over the decisions they make. Although both say they have explained their feelings to their mothers, little changes.

"We tell them, but they don't listen," Al says. "We have to listen to them or they'll disown us."

After Al underwent surgery, the two did move into an apartment together. But it was a rough go. Al liked to go out at night, playing video games at the mall and watching sporting events at local arenas. He often left Sherry home alone. She felt abandoned and alone at night. Al would stay out very late. And Sherry would worry. They toughed it out for 4 years and then finally decided that they would be happier living in separate apartments.

"Did you argue when you lived together?" a visitor asks.

"Yes," Sherry says.

"No, we did not," Al says, at nearly the same time. Then they start to argue—over whether they argued.

But they did enjoy the togetherness of living under the same roof. They would share the chores, often shopping, cleaning and cooking together.

"I liked cooking, cleaning, and passionate sex," Al says reminiscing about the good things living together had offered him.

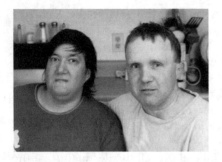

Despite the problems, the two still hold out hope that, someday, they will be able to live together as a married couple and have children. Sherry dreams of a big wedding. Since Al is Jewish and Sherry is Lutheran, they figure they would have both a pastor and a rabbi.

"We'd still want to tie the knot," Al says, but adds that both Al and Sherry's moms oppose the idea. "They said they don't think we're ready," he explains.

If they were to live together again or get married, Al says he has learned his lesson. He would do things differently. For one, he would spend more time at home—and less time carousing about. "I would spend more time with Sherry, with my Bare Feet," he says, using one of the many nicknames he has for his girlfriend.

Sherry thinks they should attend couples groups and counseling to prepare them for marriage. "No, no, no," Al objects. "We don't need that."

A flicker of nervousness passes across Sherry's kind, round face when she begins to talk about her previous relationships. She presses her lips together and remembers when she met her first boyfriend, as a teenager, living at a residential school at the other end of the state. They were friends first, but the relationship grew into something more and they decided to have sex. It was Sherry's first time. She says the two talked about their decision for a week or so before they had sex for the first time. Sherry's mother had warned her to be careful if she did have sex, to always use protection, including condoms. At Sherry's suggestion, her boyfriend went to the drugstore and bought condoms before they had sex, she remembers.

"I wasn't scared," Sherry says, waving her hands, her nails painted red, with white hearts, in honor of Valentine's Day. "I expected it to be fun and good. I talked to my mom about it. She liked Marcus's family a lot."

The two had sex for the first time when Marcus was visiting Sherry at her mother's house. It happened late at night, after her mother had gone to bed. Sherry said she was a "little surprised" at how it felt when Marcus first entered her. She also says they were both nervous.

Sherry, an only child, says that she and Marcus "almost got married." But then she left the school, after living there for 4 years, and returned to her family. "He found someone else," she says simply, no trace of regret. Other relationships were not nearly as good. She had one boyfriend who was mean. "He would say things. I finally decided I couldn't be with someone who treated me that way."

Al, Sherry says, treats her well. He helps her when she has a problem getting in touch with her counselor. He makes her laugh. And, most of all, he loves her.

Al lived at home for most of his childhood and teen years, so he had fewer opportunities to date other people. He did have one girlfriend that he met on a vacation tour with a group of other teenagers with disabilities.

"We hit it off," Al remembers, but can't recall the destination of the tour. The relationship, though, was brief. She lived a couple of hours away from Al. The two kept in touch for a few weeks, but then they drifted apart.

Al said no one ever talked to him about sex or contraception. And that was one of the reasons why he avoided having sex for many years. "I was afraid," he explains. "I didn't want to take a chance. I was afraid I might get AIDS."

With Sherry, Al felt comfortable. She was his first. The couple became sexually active soon after they started dating. Sherry had taken the contraceptive shot, Depo Provera, to prevent pregnancy.

For now, the two are content in their relationship. They see each other frequently—usually every other day. They both live alone, so there are no roommates to deal with, and they often spend the night at each other's house. They go to different events together, including a recent trip to a casino destination where Al dropped $80 in the slots. Sometimes, they go to the racetrack together in the summertime.

But, they also admit that they both like their independence and spending time away from each other, with friends or enjoying other activities. Sherry goes every Wednesday with her best friend to a group club, where they sponsor different activities, including playing games. Uno is her favorite. Al is an avid sports fan, and regularly attends sporting events. Sports is a passion Sherry shares with Al—both proudly wear their Yankees jackets—but, she isn't nearly as interested in attending events as frequently as Al is.

They have their challenges. Sherry says that "trying to get along" is the hardest part of the relationship.

"That is not true," Al fires back. "We don't fight about anything."

PAUL AND MARY

Paul lost his cat and his girlfriend in the same week. His beloved Fluffy, who had been his comforting companion since she was a kitten, died of old age. Then, Paul discovered that his girlfriend was cheating on him. He was devastated.

"It's hard when you love someone and they hurt you," Paul says.

But out of the ashes arose a second chance at love. A few months after suffering those two painful losses, Paul's social worker approached him with a proposition.

"I have a nice woman I want you to meet," she told Paul.

At first, he was excited. But then the social worker revealed that the mystery woman was Mary, his ex-girlfriend's roommate. Paul was wary.

"I said, 'Are you crazy?'" he remembers now, about 15 years later. He didn't think that he and Mary would make a good match. Plus, there was the baggage of her being his ex-girlfriend's roommate. But, after thinking about it, Paul decided to give it a try.

"I said, 'We'll see how it works, but I ain't promising you nothing.'"

The couple recently celebrated their 10th anniversary. Paul bought Mary a beautiful diamond ring, 14 karat gold with baguettes decorating each side of the center diamond. Mary holds out her hand, displaying the ring that is a sign of the love that has kept the two together through job changes, apartment moves, and the ups and downs of daily living.

"She's got a good heart and all that," says Paul, 46, a stocky man with a crew cut and salt and pepper hair.

"He's a good looking man," Mary, 52, says of her husband. "He's got a great personality. He made me laugh."

When they first started dating, Paul and Mary would share a small single bed in the apartment where Mary lived. Mary remembers the first time they had sex. It was like getting even closer to a good friend. "I wasn't scared," she says. "I knew Paul was a gentle man." They only used condoms the first couple of times, they said. Because of Mary's age, they did not feel that pregnancy was a risk. Neither wanted children.

They dated for several years before Paul proposed to Mary in the office of the Burger King where he worked for 15 years.

"I felt you can't live alone forever," Paul says, explaining his reasons for wanting to marry. "You need somebody around to talk to and things, so that's why."

"I was excited," Mary remembers. "I said yes right away. I called my mother. She was so happy for us. She started making the arrangements right away."

The couple exchanged wedding vows with 275 family and friends in attendance. Their wedding photo sits on the end table in their spacious living room, its pink frame faded from the years. They've lived for about 5 years in the handsome three-bedroom brick-front home. They even have a new cat—Nemo. Paul describes his job at Burger King. "I'm a burger flipper," he says. Mary sometimes cares for a friend's children, while the parents work. They've both settled into the ebb and flow of their daily lives and rarely argue over anything major, they say.

"We don't have any really big fights," Paul says. "Sometimes I give in, if it's over something stupid. After we have a quarrel, and I think about it, I'll say, 'I didn't mean to yell, but you aggravated the heck out of me.'"

Mary had several boyfriends over the years, but she says she was never sexually active with any of them. She dated one man for 6 years, but found out that he was cheating on her. "I saw him cheating and just stopped seeing him," she says.

Like Lorraine, Mary's first sexual encounter was forced. When she was about 20 years old, Mary was raped by the son of the woman who operated the boarding house where Mary was living. The woman had left for the afternoon. And her son forced himself on her.

"It was scary," Mary remembers.

Luckily, Mary had taken sexuality education classes while at a training school, where she had learned about rape. "They talked about sexual assault," Mary explains. "That's how I knew it was wrong when I was raped."

After the rape, Mary immediately called her parents. Her father picked her up and took her to the hospital. The police were called. A restraining order was issued against the man. But he was never prosecuted. His mother sided with her son, denying that he had been alone with Mary. It was Mary's word against her attacker. The matter was dropped.

Shortly after, Mary became a member of her current support agency. The organization helped her find her own studio apartment. It was the first time she had her own place and she has been living on her own ever since.

Paul's parents died when he was young. He and his brother were sent to live with another, older brother, but this brother and wife had marital problems and were unable to continue caring for Paul and his brother. The state placed the children in a shelter, where they lived for 3 years. A family adopted his younger brother. Paul was placed in an institution, where he lived for 7 years. He was released to the community when he was in his early 20s.

For 30 years, Paul never saw his brother. The two grew up and led their own lives, never knowing where the other was, but also always remembering the close bond they had shared. A few years ago, a niece arranged a reunion of the long-lost brothers. It was a special moment in Paul's life, and Mary was happy to share it with him. Now, they regularly visit Paul's brother's family, and Mary has grown close to this newfound family.

"His brother fell in love with me," she says.

The two also regularly visit with other family members, including a passel of nieces and nephews, whose pictures are scattered around their home.

So, what's the best part of being married?

"You know, I've been asking myself that question for the longest time," Paul quips.

But then he grows more serious. "Growing old together," he says. "Having a companion and a partner." Mary nods and takes her husband's hand. "Growing old together. That's the best thing."

So in the end, these couples are not all that different from the millions of people who fall in love, fumble through the difficulties of loving and living with another person and who try to make it work. If they are lucky, they will find a peaceful place next to the person they love. A place they can stay forever.

7

Cultural Diversity, Sexuality Education, and Intellectual Disability

Ruth Luckasson and Sherry Niccolai

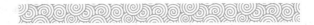

Children, youth, and adults with intellectual disabilities, like their peers with other types of disabilities and without disabilities, live in a culturally diverse world. Cultural diversity, which adds layers of richness to one's life, can also challenge communication and relationships between individuals. Sexuality, which is strongly rooted in communication and relationships, can thus be both enriched and challenged by cultural diversity. It is critical for individuals with intellectual disabilities, their families, friends, teachers, and support staff to consider culture when communicating about sexuality, attempting to understand relationships, and planning and delivering sexuality education.

This chapter addresses the issues of culture as they affect sexuality education for people with intellectual disabilities. We focus on ethnic culture rather than disability culture, which, although also critical, is beyond the scope of this chapter (see, e.g., Gill, 1995). The purpose of the chapter is to increase understanding of the role of ethnic culture in communicating about sexuality, understanding and improving relationships, teaching about sexuality, and enhancing the richness of the lives people with intellectual disabilities create for themselves.

The chapter is organized around the following questions: What is culture? What is the place of culture in the lives of people with intellectual disabilities? How does culture affect sexuality for individuals with disabilities? How should sexuality education reflect culture? How might an educator make decisions about what and how to teach? How should one address cultural differences between students and teachers? How might one avoid cultural stereotypes?

WHAT IS CULTURE?

According to pioneering anthropologist Edward T. Hall (1976), culture is

> the total communication framework: words, actions, postures, gestures, tones of voice, facial expressions, the way he[/she] handles time, space, and materials, and the way he[/she] works, plays, *makes love,* and defends himself[/herself]. All these things and more are complete communication systems with meanings that can be read correctly only if one is familiar with the behavior in its historical, social and cultural context. (p. 42; emphasis added)

Culture permeates everything—how we think, speak, act, look, feel, and live. The genuine meaning of any human behavior can be understood only if one is sensitive to the cultural context of the thinking, speaking, acting, looking, feeling, and living of the other person. Individuals of different cultures can communicate and understand each other if they are willing to understand each others' cultures. But people often make serious cultural mistakes—usually through ignorance or by making assumptions based on their own culture and ignoring or devaluing other people's cultures. These cultural mistakes can cause significant problems, ranging from mixed signals to hurt feelings to anger and humiliation, or even criminal violations or international disasters. It is important that a sexuality educator avoid making cultural errors, and it is also important that the sexuality educator assist an individual with intellectual disabilities to avoid serious cultural mistakes in the area of sexual expression.

WHAT IS THE PLACE OF CULTURE IN THE LIVES OF PEOPLE WITH INTELLECTUAL DISABILITIES?

The cultural diversity of individuals with disabilities has often been denied or ignored. Individuals have been assumed to have either no culture because they were "too disabled" to understand anything related to culture, or they have had to take on the culture of their current support staff or residential placement and abandon expression of their own culture. This has led to routine denial of an important part of the humanity of each individual: their cultural identity, and perhaps even their language (de Valenzuela & Niccolai, 2004).

Behavior must be understood within the context of culture (Hall, 1976). And the extent to which any individual has "acculturated" to the dominant culture varies by the individual (Collier, 1998). In the past, the culture (and stage of acculturation) of many individuals with disabilities was ignored, with negative consequences to the individual. Individuals who had grown up in an English-speaking family, for example, might be placed into a residential setting in which all support providers spoke another language and functioned as in another culture; individuals who immigrated from another country and only spoke the language of that country were often diagnosed with a disability solely on the basis of their inability to speak English; actions appropriate in a home culture could be severely punished in the unfamiliar culture; and individuals with disabilities whose first language was not English were frequently deprived of opportunities to communicate in their first language and also deprived of instruction to learn English.

Individuals with intellectual disabilities are members of their own culture and also live in a culturally diverse world. Increased educational inclusion and community integrated living and working broaden their experiences with others (Wehmeyer, Sands, Knowlton, & Kozleski, 2002). Each person with intellectual disabilities experiences communication and relationships through his or her own culture and likely relates to several people of other cultures daily. Consider the following hypothetical example:

Sharon is a middle-age woman with an intellectual ability who immigrated in the 1940s as a child to the United States from Germany with her now-deceased parents. Sharon lived with her parents in a rural German-American farming community until her parents died when she was 40 years old. She then moved to a large Midwestern city to be nearer to her sister. Sharon currently lives in her own urban home with a female roommate who grew up in an East Coast inner city. They are supported by a culturally diverse staff, including an older woman who emigrated from Laos 20 years ago, a young man who recently arrived from central Africa, and a middle-age Caucasian Mennonite volunteer.

Sharon works as part of a crew of people with intellectual disabilities that contracts to provide cleaning services to several neighborhood ethnic restaurants. Her man friend, Joseph, who is Hispanic, also works on the crew. Sharon and Joseph belong to a social group facilitated by a social worker, Amy, who teaches about many aspects of adult living, including relationship and sexuality education. Sharon and Joseph get together each weekend for social activities, and they would like to get married and have a child in the future.

Think about the rich cultural diversity in Sharon's life. How might culture affect Sharon's communication and relationships? Might there be potential cultural misunderstandings between Sharon and the people in her life? What should Amy consider when providing relationship and sexuality education to Sharon and the other members of the group?

HOW DOES CULTURE AFFECT SEXUALITY FOR INDIVIDUALS WITH DISABILITIES?

Edgerton described tremendous variety in the ways that different cultures have treated the sexuality of individuals with intellectual disabilities (Edgerton, 1970). He wrote of the Vietnamese Amman in which even individuals with severe disabilities were allowed to marry and inherit property (citing Thompson, 1937); certain parts of India in which the legality of a marriage required court adjudication (citing Mayne, 1953); areas of East Africa and Bali in which people with intellectual disabilities were denied access to *any* sexual expression (citing Wilson, 1963; Covarrubias, 1938); and highland societies in New Guinea in which women, but not men, with intellectual disabilities had the opportunity for marriage (citing Oosterwal, 1961). After 35 years, the world has changed and cultures have changed, but incredible diversity remains.

For each person with intellectual disabilities, the following aspects of sexuality might be affected by their culture:

- Recognition of and preparation for sexual maturity
- Communication style
- Personal values
- Construction of social cues
- Determination of what is sexually acceptable and what is taboo
- Courtship practices
- Expectations of acceptable behavior by men and women
- Assumptions of certain adult roles
- Relationships to parents
- Designation of violating or criminal behavior
- Marriage practices
- The place of children in a family

Thus, sexuality education must consider the culture of the person. Moreover, in addition to the culture of the person receiving education, the culture of friends, family, the community, and even the culture of the individual providing the education must be considered.

Ricky's story demonstrates some of the complex ways in which culture might affect sexuality.

> Ricky is a teenage Native American youth with intellectual disabilities who was adopted as an adolescent by an Anglo-dominant culture family after an automobile accident killed his biological family. Ricky's new family loves him deeply and tries to be nonjudgmental about cultural differences. They consider themselves a sexually liberated family and have frequent lengthy family conversations about all aspects of sexuality. They state that they are encouraging Ricky to be more open about his sexuality. Ricky is extremely uncomfortable in these conversations, but he is grateful to his adoptive family and does not want to offend them. For Ricky, sexuality is a very private topic in his culture, and he believes that its expression should be limited to procreation and not pursued for pleasure alone. He reacts to the family conversations by hiding his eyes, posturally withdrawing, cringing, and never challenging his family, even though he is deeply shamed by having to participate in these conversations. His adoptive family noticed his behavior and attributes it to unnecessary shyness. The family has not spoken with Ricky about his culture's beliefs about sexuality, nor have they asked tribal leaders or others who might have relevant knowledge. They state they are "helping Ricky become more comfortable with his sexuality." Ricky has begun to consider running away from home in order to escape his discomfort.

What has gone wrong in Ricky's situation? Which steps have been missed? How might the family and Ricky step back and attempt to repair this situation?

HOW SHOULD SEXUALITY EDUCATION REFLECT CULTURE?

It is ironic that the two areas that are often ignored in the education of people with intellectual disabilities are sexuality education and culturally competent teaching. Sexuality education should be culturally competent or culturally reciprocal (and should meet the standards set forth in this book in other chapters). Cultural reciprocity refers to a process of learning about a person and his or her family, talking with them about the assumptions that underlie their cultural values and priorities, reflecting on one's own cultural values and priorities, analyzing potential conflicts, and sharing and adapting to the person's culture and values (Harry & Kalyanpur, 1999). Communication is a key to this reciprocity.

Rogers and Steinfatt (1999) explained the complexities of intercultural communication competence; the effective and appropriate exchange of information between individuals who are different culturally. They urged increased recognition and respect of different ways of thinking.

What constitutes culturally sensitive sexuality education planning for individuals with intellectual disabilities? It is important that a sexuality educator consider these important steps when developing a culturally appropriate sexuality education plan.

- Know the laws and regulations of the jurisdiction and agency
- Know the ethical requirements and standards of your profession
- Learn about the student's culture and the ways it affects sexuality
- Reflect on your own culture and the way it affects you
- Communicate about the sexuality learning objectives and negotiate an individualized plan that respects culture
- Periodically review and revise the plan

Sexuality education must be consistent with any legal requirements of the jurisdiction. A sexuality educator must be cognizant of any laws and regulations of the state and agency of his or her location and must follow those laws. In addition, educators must know the ethics and standards of the profession and follow those standards.

Sexuality planning must also be individually determined and student focused. This means that the concept of student-centered planning, focusing on the desired personal outcomes of an individual and coordinating the resources necessary to implement those outcomes, requires that both sexuality and cultural diversity be addressed. If one important purpose of education is to prepare individuals to create personally satisfying lives for themselves, it is essential for individuals to develop knowledge of sexuality and the ability to function in their diverse communities. As Duh (1999) stated, "Individuals with disabilities can be successfully integrated into the general community because they can be armed through special education and training with acceptable skills involved in social interaction, self-care, and daily living" (p. 302). Part of the idea of integration into a community should certainly involve an understanding of one's sexuality and the development of skills to develop appropriate relationships and avoid inappropriate relationships.

A sexuality educator should learn as much as possible about a student's culture and the ways it might affect the student. And, the educator must reflect on his or her own culture and how that culture affects his or her attitudes, beliefs, and behaviors. From this deep level of understanding of both the student's and the educator's cultures, they should negotiate (while considering legal, regulatory, ethical, and standards-based authority) a plan that respects the student's culture. Finally, any plan should be well documented in writing and periodically reviewed and revised.

HOW MIGHT AN EDUCATOR MAKE
DECISIONS ABOUT WHAT AND HOW TO TEACH?

Access to sexuality education for individuals with intellectual disabilities will require modifications. What modifications are required to address culture? Some argue that translating a sexuality education into another language for a culturally different student is the only change needed. Mere translation, however, does not address the critical issues of culture. It's not just the words that must be understood, but the total communication framework described by Hall (1976). This is similar to the debate about whether it is more important to assimilate or to accommodate. Certainly, it might be easier for educators to assume a cookie-cutter teaching style that treats all students exactly the same and assumes that they all have the same culture, life experiences, and goals as the educator and need to have the "cookie-cutter" curriculum simply translated into another language. However, this ethnocentric attitude undermines human dignity, effective teaching, and learning. Teachers striving to create a student-centered curriculum need to consider each actual student, in all his or her individuality.

> Consider the cultural negotiation that might be required in order to develop a community integration, relationship, and sexuality education plan for a female teenager who is Muslim. What would you want to know about her culture and how would you learn? Suppose the only existing transition work settings are coeducational, and the teen and her family refuse to permit any coeducational aspects of a plan? One of your colleagues at the school tells you that you should report their refusal as "educational neglect" under the mandatory reporting requirements of the state child protective services law. What do you do?

A student's daily life must be considered when preparing a student-centered lesson. Often, people with disabilities live with their family members. If they need assistance or care, it is frequently family members who provide that care. Their social group is likely made up of family, immediate and extended, and community, which often reflect the ethnic background of the family.

Consider a Mexican man with intellectual disabilities, living in Albuquerque, New Mexico, who is more a part of the Mexican community than the Anglo community. When teaching this man social skills and an understanding of social opportunities, it is important to remember where and with whom he will use these skills. It is simply not logical for a student to receive sexuality education based solely on the dominant Anglo culture of the United States if the dominant Anglo culture is not the only part, or even largest part, of his daily life.

A familiar example would be greeting another person. If this man were to attend a sexuality education class based on dominant Anglo culture, he might learn that it is inappropriate to kiss people he has just met. However, in Mexican culture, a kiss on the cheek is a common greeting between men and women. What may be good information for his Anglo classmates living solely in Anglo cultures has just become misinformation for this Mexican man. His needs must be considered in the planning—where is his social life? With whom is he spending time? Does he need to learn to function in more than one culture?

If the goal of education is to prepare a person for his or her life, then the person's life must be considered when planning.

When modifying a curriculum, an educator might consider changing the selection of learning objectives, the amount of time designated to teach different aspects of sexuality education, the vocabulary, and the potential joys, responsibilities, and risks. For example, understanding inappropriate attention is especially important for people with intellectual disabilities. The rate of abuse against individuals with mental retardation is higher than in typically developing people (McCurry, McClellan, & Adams, 1998). Attackers look for "good victims," those that may be perceived as weaker and, therefore, easier targets. People with disabilities may be seen as a better target by a victimizer and, therefore, need information to protect themselves from potential abuse.

Abuse must not be seen as something that is committed only by strangers, however. And segregation, even if legal, is not the answer. Abuse has occurred in segregated settings and by "safe" people such as family members, religious figures, or authorities (Nicol, 1998; Pound, 1996; Sobsey, 1995). Additionally, the loneliness individuals with intellectual disabilities may feel and the savvy they may lack due to their isolation may actually increase their vulnerability to an abuser who may have entered their lives as a "safe" person. Therefore, explicit instruction on what is and what is not appropriate behavior is a necessary part of sexuality education for individuals with intellectual disabilities. Isolating individuals does not protect them from abuse—education and social supports are more effective protection.

Protection from abuse and enhancement of life will vary based on culture. McCabe (as cited in Bambury, 1999) stated: "Research indicates that people with mild intellectual disability are likely to need special help if they are to acquire socially appropriate sexual behavior, to make safe sexual choices, and to become less vulnerable to sexual abuse from others in the community" (p. 207). Instruction about socially appropriate sexual behavior as well as protection from victimization will need to consider the actual culture and community of the individual.

Social status, family, peers, and community are major factors in the development of identity and views of sexuality (Huerta-Franco & Malacara, 1999; Lunsky & Mary, 1998; "Special section: Sexuality and ethnicity, part II," 1997). But, as Garwood (2000) urged, sexuality education must prepare people for "real life situations" (p. 280). A person's "real life" must be what guides their sexuality education program.

> Consider the case of Sara, an African American middle-age woman with intellectual disabilities who has lived all her life in the rural South. When Sara was deinstitutionalized from a Southern institution last year, her planning team considered where she should live. She has one uncle who lives in California, so Sara moved to a large California city where her uncle lives so that she could be close to a family member. The team decided that because of her skin color she would live with a black foster family and be assigned a black social worker. So, Sara moved in with a family that emigrated from a Caribbean island 5 years ago, and her social worker is a woman from Congo who received her professional training in England. Recently, the supervisor at Sara's work site raised concerns about possible abuse. Sara stated that she "sleeps with the family so they can wake me up." The work supervisor has asked the sexuality educator to "do something." How might culture affect this case?

Some would argue that it doesn't matter what cultures are represented in the learning situation, if individuals are in the United States, they need to learn to do things the "American way." First, it is necessary to emphasize that regardless of ethnic affiliation, the laws of the United States must be followed by all who live and work within the jurisdiction or otherwise come within the arm of the law. In addition, if a student has contact with the dominant U.S. culture, it is certainly important to give him or her the tools necessary to function well within that culture. However, teaching students how to act appropriately in Anglo culture to the exclusion of their own, or vice versa, is a tremendous disservice. If students are bicultural, as are most culturally diverse people in the world, they need to know how to navigate both societies, and this includes providing them with a sexuality education program that addresses the differences in their cultures. Educators cannot make a political protest of diversity by teaching culturally and linguistically diverse students how to be "Americans" without doing a serious disservice to those students. Ignoring their cultural backgrounds and culturally based funds of knowledge will create confusion and misinformation for these students.

CULTURAL DIFFERENCES
BETWEEN STUDENTS AND TEACHERS

A dilemma may occur when the culture of a student and the culture of the educator are in conflict in a certain area of sexuality education. For example, if sexual harassment (by American legal definition) is something that is tolerated, expected, and seen as harmless in a student's home culture, the educator has to make a decision about how to deal with the discrepancy. Certainly, the educator has an obligation to help the individual avoid actions that violate local law or human rights.

International business has been confronted with a similar conflict, although outside of the physical borders of the United States. Global companies have found themselves in situations in which foreign offices were violating sexual harassment and discrimination policies of the home U.S. office. Companies that tried to take action were in a difficult situation. They ultimately determined that they could not apply U.S. standards of harassment to a different jurisdiction. Although it might be tempting, a person cannot force his or her belief system upon another group. Instead, for businesses, the rules of conduct for offices outside of the United States were based on local laws and culture (Maatman, 2000). This example, while illustrative of the tension, is limited to situations outside of the United States.

It is important that sexuality education does not become a place to impose the individual educator's culturally-based sense of correctness, but rather a place to teach students to develop the necessary skills to live law-abiding, happy, and safe lives with respect to their own activities and community. This must be balanced, however, with respect for the laws of the jurisdiction.

Missy, age 11, has a significant intellectual disability. Her teacher repeatedly refers to Missy as her "baby." When Missy began to have menstrual periods, her teacher and the sexuality educator at her school told her that she should keep it private and not talk about it. Missy became confused and upset. In her Native American culture, the community holds a celebration when a girl has her first menstrual period. Not only do people talk about it amongst themselves, they also hold a big community event in honor of the occasion. Everyone comes out to celebrate the girl's newly mature status and her valued ability to contribute to the community by bearing children. Behavioral expectations also dramatically change with the girl's new status—physical contact or time alone with males, including brothers and other family members, is strictly forbidden. Also, the girl should no longer play or engage in juvenile activities with boys. Missy cannot reconcile the embarrassment and infantalization she experiences at school with the community celebration in honor of her new maturity she experienced at home.

AVOIDING CULTURAL STEREOTYPES

How should the content of sexuality education be modified for cultural groups? Although this may seem like a relatively simple question, the answer is quite complex. Without making generalizations, which could ultimately lead to stereotypes, it is difficult to say that there is one specific way to teach sexuality education to a given ethnic group. Like Americans, most groups are diverse. People from the same ethnic background may be very different due to life experiences, age, religion, or degree of acculturation into the dominant culture. When teaching diverse students, it is important to remember that differences in their behaviors, attitudes, experiences, and opinions might be due to cultural differences and not abuse or misinformation. Therefore, educators need to develop tools to differentiate between normal and unusual behavior within a culture.

Consider, for example, the case of Carla, a young Chinese woman. It would be overgeneralizing to assume that "all Chinese believe X about sexuality." Carla's culture may be influenced by traditional Confucianism, which "demands that a woman be obedient to her father, husband, and son and to cultivate chastity, speech, artistry, and demeanor" (Weizhen, 1985, p. 54). The Chinese Cultural Revolution and contemporary beliefs about equality of the sexes may also influence Carla's beliefs. In addition, it is likely that Carla's behavior and relationships will be highly affected by her family. "In Chinese society, interpersonal relationships cannot be removed from the influence of the family" (Xintian, 1985, p. 90). Thus, individualization and student-centered planning are the keys to understanding how Carla's culture influences her sexuality education.

Certain aspects of a sexuality education program can be said to be more culturally based than others. Anatomy, for example could be said to have more of a base in biology than culture. How it is taught, however, as well as what discussions, activities, and pictures are taboo, is cultural (Williams, personal communication, July 8, 2002). Also, aspects such as gender roles can vary greatly from one culture to another

(Flaskerud, Uman, & Lara, 1996; Mutua & Dimitrov, 2001; "Special section: Sexuality and ethnicity, part II," 1997). In addition, long-term goals, such as what an appropriate adult life is like for individuals with and without disabilities are also culturally based (Matteson, 1997; Mutua & Dimitrov, 2001).

Expressions of sexuality can also vary tremendously. Some cultures, for example, do not allow homosexuality to be acknowledged openly (Flaskerud et al., 1996; Matteson, 1997; Relic, 2001). Fudon University in Shanghai, China recently launched China's first undergraduate course on gay and lesbian studies (French, 2005). However, it can also be said of some cultures that sexuality in general, regardless of preference, is something to be treated with intense privacy (Matteson, 1997). Shame, as well as what is considered shameful, is certainly a culturally based phenomenon (Yang & Rosenblatt, 2001).

Sexual harassment is not defined worldwide as it is in the United States. Even the laws of other countries do not necessarily agree with the U.S. legal system on what constitutes harassment (Conway, 1998). Certain cultures in Latin America, for example, regularly engage in behavior that would be considered harassment by U.S. standards. Even something that may seem as universal as the taboo against incest is cultural (Gilman, 1998). For example, the Navajo people of the southwestern United States base family identification on not one, but four clans. Sexual contact with any person that shares any one of those four clans is considered an incestuous relationship. A well-intentioned educator without knowledge of the Navajo clan system who encourages such a relationship could enable an act that in Navajo culture is no less serious than an educator enabling a sexual relationship between cousins in Anglo society (Aronilth, 1992).

HOW CAN AN EDUCATOR MAKE DECISIONS?

Obviously, no educator can expect to know every culture intimately. In addition, just as Americans cannot be defined by one morality, or one set of guidelines, it is difficult to develop a set of cultural rules for another group without inaccurate stereotyping. Perhaps the best way to get information is to talk with students, parents, or family members. If the parents or family is not available, then other members of the community can become cultural informants. It is absolutely necessary for educators to accept that they cannot know all of the answers about cultural diversity with respect to sexuality, and that the most important thing may be to know when to ask for help and who can be a reliable cultural informant. However, it is necessary to remember that there is always variation within a culture, just as there is within what is considered "American." As a Mennonite family in rural Pennsylvania will have different views about their child's sexuality than a liberal family in Berkeley, California, so too will there be diversity within any labeled group. Cultural informants, while valuable, may not always have much in common with the student. For this reason, if possible, family members should be directly involved as much as possible in the planning stages to ensure that the information presented is culturally relevant. In addition, it is with information gathered in the community and family that an educator can evaluate a person's behavior with respect to culture. What may seem like inappropriate affection to an educator might be perfectly normal behavior for a student within his or her community.

Another difficulty in modifying sexuality education for culturally diverse students is the overgeneralizing of cultural groups that has already occurred. Two major groups of the Southwest part of the United States, Hispanics and Native Americans, have tremendous variation within them, yet each is often seen as one homogenous entity. The term *Hispanic* covers people from all socioeconomic levels and a tremendous variety of cultures. In fact, what links Hispanics more than anything is a common language. The cultures found in Cuba, Mexico, Argentina, and the United States, although incredibly different, are all found under the umbrella term of *Hispanic.* Although linguistically they may be similar, culturally they cannot be said to be the same. Sexuality, like other aspects of culture, varies greatly within Hispanic cultures. Torres and Cernada (2003) reported many intra-Hispanic differences related to important issues such as sexual negotiation, balance of power between men and women, accepted age of marriage, accepted age of first pregnancy and whether teenage parenthood is stigmatized, number of pregnancies and who determines the number, duration of breastfeeding, acceptance of medical prenatal care versus more personal interventions by members of the community, and incorporation of beliefs about therapeutic use of music, poetry, and drama. Clearly, a sexuality educator must genuinely explore cultural influences while avoiding overgeneralizing or stereotyping about "Hispanic sexuality."

Native Americans also find themselves grouped together, irrespective of the variation that is found in the more than 550 federally recognized tribes in the United States (Native American Rights Fund, 2004). In addition, religion, traditionalism, degree of acculturation, lifestyle, and other factors will affect the formation of their sexuality to such a degree that a "Native American based" sexuality education program would be too broad to provide individuals with the specific information that they need to design programs to help students face real life situations in their home communities.

Geographic location as well as diversity of the area should be considered. If individuals have interactions with members of other ethnic groups, it is certainly logical and important to give them the social skills to interact appropriately with members of that group. Multicultural education should not be reserved solely for students who are themselves culturally diverse, but should also be made available for students who have interactions with members of other ethnic groups (that is, *all* students).

CONCLUSION

Culture is the total communication framework of a human being. The culture of each individual with intellectual disabilities is a critical consideration in planning and providing sexuality education. An educator cannot be an expert in the culture of every person he or she teaches. However, an educator should have the right tools to gain an understanding of elements of a culture that are necessary to any educational plan. Cultural competence and effective intercultural communication are critical. The best sources of information are individuals, their families, and members of their communities. Talking directly with them will allow an educator to develop a clearer picture of a student's culture, daily life, and expected behaviors instead of teaching to a stereotyped idea or forcing the student to totally conform to a culture that is not his or her own. Sexuality is rooted in communication and relationships, and communication and relationship are rooted in culture.

REFERENCES

Aronilth, W., Jr. (1992). *Foundation of Navajo culture*. Tsaile, AZ: Tsaile Press.

Bambury, J. (1999). Effects of two experimental educational programs on the socio-sexual knowledge and attitudes of adults with mild intellectual disability. *Education and Training in Mental Retardation and Developmental Disabilities, 34*(2), 207–211.

Collier, C. (1998). *Separating difference from disability: Assessing diverse learners.* Ferndale, WA: Cross-Cultural Developmental Education Services.

Conway, M.E. (1998). Sexual harassment abroad. *Workforce, 3*(5), 8–9.

de Valenzuela, J.S., & Niccolai, S. (2004). Language development in culturally and linguistically diverse students with special education needs. In L.M. Baca & H.T. Cervantes (Eds.), *The bilingual special education interface* (4th ed., pp. 124–161). Upper Saddle River, NJ: Pearson/Merrill Prentice Hall.

Duh, J. (1999). Sexual knowledge, attitudes, and experiences of high school students with and without disabilities in Taiwan. *Education and Training in Mental Retardation and Developmental Disabilities, 34*(3), 302–311.

Edgerton, R.B. (1970). Mental retardation in non-Western societies: Toward a cross-cultural perspective on incompetence. In H.C. Haywood (Ed.), *Social-cultural aspects of mental retardation* (pp. 523–559). New York: Meredith.

Flaskerud, J.H., Uman, G., & Lara, R. (1996). Sexual practices, attitudes and knowledge related to HIV transmission in low income Los Angeles Hispanic women. *The Journal of Sexual Research, 33*(4), 343–353.

French, H.W. (2005, Sept. 8). A Chinese university removes a topic from the closet. *The New York Times,* p. A3.

Garwood, M. (2000). Impact of sexual education programs on sexual knowledge and feelings of men with a mild intellectual disability. *Education and Training in Mental Retardation and Developmental Disabilities, 35*(3), 269–283.

Gill, C. (1995, fall). A psychological view of disability culture. *Disabilities Studies Quarterly.* Retrieved November 13, 2005, from http://www.independentliving .org/docs3/gill1995.html

Gilman, S.L. (1998). Sibling incest, madness, and the "Jews." *Social Research, 65*(2), 401–433.

Hall, E.T. (1976). *Beyond culture.* New York: Doubleday.

Harry, B., & Kalyanpur, M. (1999). *Culture in special education.* Baltimore: Paul H. Brookes Publishing Co.

Huerta-Franco, R., & Malacara, J.M. (1999). Factors associated with the sexual experiences of underprivileged Mexican adolescents. *Adolescence, 34*(134), 389–401.

Lunsky, Y.J., & Mary, K.M. (1998). The attitudes of individuals with autism and mental retardation towards sexuality. *Education and Training in Mental Retardation and Developmental Disabilities, 33*(1), 24–33.

Maatman, G.L., Jr. (2000). A global view of sexual harassment. *HR Magazine, 45*(7), 151–158.

Matteson, D.R. (1997). Bisexual and homosexual behavior and HIV risk among Chinese-American, Filipino-, and Korean-American men. *The Journal of Sexual Research, 34*(1), 93–104.

McCurry, C., McClellan, J.M., & Adams, J. (1998). Sexual behavior associated with low verbal IQ in youth who have severe mental illness. *Mental Retardation, 36,* 23–30.

Mutua, N.K., & Dimitrov, D.M. (2001). Parents' expectations about future outcomes of children with mental retardation in Kenya: Differential effects of gender and severity of mental retardation. *The Journal of Special Education, 35*(3), 172–180.

Native American Rights Fund. (2004). *Annual Report.* Retrieved November 13, 2005, from http://www.narf.org/pubs/ar/NARF2004.pdf

Nicol, J. (1998). Mystery at Gagetown. *Maclean's, 111*(28), 22–24.

Pound, E.T. (1996). Faith, death and betrayal. *U.S. News & World Report, 120,* 42–48.

Relic, P.D. (2001). The new wisdom in sexuality education. *Independent School, 60*(2), 7–8.

Rogers, E.M., & Steinfatt, T.M. (1999). *Intercultural communication.* Prospect Heights, IL: Waveland.

Sobsey, D. (1995). *Violence and abuse in the lives of people with disabilities: An end of silent acceptance?* Baltimore: Paul H. Brookes Publishing Co.

Special section: Sexuality and ethnicity, part II. (1997). *The Journal of Sexual Research, 34*(1), 67–111.

Torres, M.I., & Cernada, G.P. (2003). *Sexual and reproductive health promotion in Latino populations: Parteras, promotoras, and poetas: Case studies.* Amityville, NY: Baywood.

Wehmeyer, M.L., Sands, D.J., Knowlton, H.E., & Kozleski, E.B. (2002). The emergent self: Sexuality and social inclusion. In *Teaching students with mental retardation: Providing access to the general curriculum* (pp. 204–217). Baltimore: Paul H. Brookes Publishing Co.

Weizhen, S. (1985). A preliminary study of the character traits of the Chinese. In W.S. Tseng & D.Y.H. Wu (Eds.), *Chinese culture and mental health* (pp. 47–55). Orlando, FL: Academic Press.

Xintian, L. (1985). The effect of family on the mental health of the Chinese people. In W.S. Tseng & D.Y.H. Wu (Eds.), *Chinese culture and mental health* (pp. 85–93). Orlando, FL: Academic Press.

Yang, S., & Rosenblatt, P.C. (2001). Shame in Korean families. *Journal of Comparative Family Studies, 32*(3), 361–375.

8

Supporting Diversity
in Sexual Relationships

On Being Gay, Lesbian, Bisexual, or
Transgender with an Intellectual Disability

John D. Allen

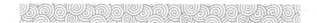

The Rainbow Support Group (RSG) is a unique group providing support and affirmation for people with intellectual and other developmental disabilities who are gay, lesbian, bisexual, and transgender (GLBT). The group, which began in September 1998 at the New Haven Gay & Lesbian Community Center in New Haven, Connecticut, is shattering the myths and stereotypes surrounding people with mental retardation. Not only are people with these disabilities full human beings with the same needs and desires for intimacy and healthy sexual expression as people without intellectual disabilities, but the group is evidence that some people with an intellectual or developmental disability or mental retardation have an understanding of sexual orientation as well.

"How do they know?" is a frequent question from people both within and outside of the profession when they first hear about the RSG. The question is at once innocent and insulting—an indictment of the patronizing regard society has of people with intellectual and developmental disabilities.

How does someone with an intellectual or developmental disability know that he or she is gay? The same way someone else with an intellectual or developmental disability knows that he or she is heterosexual. It is as simple as *they just do,* by paying attention to what is going on inside of them (Marcus, 1993).

Members of the RSG came to know they were part of the sexual minority community the same way anyone else comes to a GLBT support group. Their stories of coming out are similar to other gay people. The awareness typically occurs over time, as the vignettes of life begin to reveal a sexual understanding different from the majority. People with intellectual or developmental disabilities or mental retardation know that they are gay by being in touch with their feelings, through sexual experimentation, and, hopefully, by participating in a shared community.

Many members of the RSG speak of an early awareness of their sexual orientation, which is known as their "coming-out" experience. Most of the members, who are now between the ages of 30 and 50, describe their coming out experiences as occurring between 10–15 years of age, compared with typically developing peers, who came out in their mid- to late twenties (Marcus, 1993).

WE'RE HERE, WE'RE QUEER: WHAT IS THE GAY COMMUNITY?

The *gay community* is an inclusive term that refers to disparate groups bound together by their separateness (Marcus, 1993). The gay community generally includes gay men, lesbian women, and people who identify as bisexual and transgender (Gay & Lesbian Alliance Against Defamation [GLAAD], 2001). The term *gay* has a dual meaning. It can be used to identify homosexual men, but is also an easy term to refer to the entire GLBT community (GLAAD, 2001).

Transgender is an umbrella term that refers to people that cross-dress, including males that wear feminine clothing and females that wear masculine clothing (GLAAD, 2001). It also includes people that are in various stages of having gender reassignment surgery to become transsexual (GLAAD, 2001). An individual who identifies as transgender, however, does not have to be gay. The RSG, for example, includes a 55-year-old man who identifies as heterosexual, has a girlfriend, and yet has cross-dressed throughout his life.

A bisexual person is someone who can be sexually attracted to both men and women (Marcus, 1993). In addition, for some people, identifying as a bisexual person can seem more culturally acceptable than making a declaration as an exclusively gay or lesbian person. Certainly some members of the RSG, who are acutely aware of social stigma associated with their disability, may find it easier to first identify as bisexual and then over time declare exclusivity as they feel more comfortable being connected to the gay community. However, some members have remained consistent that they are attracted to both men and women. What has become clear is that navigating the coming out process is complicated for people with intellectual or developmental disabilities or mental retardation, and is made even more so since they face additional obstacles to self-advocacy.

The RSG was invited by YAI, formerly known as the Young Adult Institute, a large provider of services for individuals with disabilities and a developer of many training materials for staff and program participants, to speak at their International Conference in New York City in 2000. During this trip, RSG's first, the members were adamant about taking a side trip to Greenwich Village following the afternoon presentation. The members remembered with remarkably vivid detail the historical discussions of the early gay movement and wanted to visit the Stonewall Café, which is credited as the birthplace of the modern gay movement. The members remain incredulous at knowing that on the last weekend of June in 1969 a group of drag queens, butch lesbians, and other social outcasts raged against a routine police raid and kicked off a three day rebellion that signaled the beginning of a modern gay sensibility (Duberman, 1993). There is a sense of power in knowing the tribulations of gay people from previous generations. They know, too, the significance of the RSG as a pioneer group that is making visible a minority within a minority.

THE TIME HAS COME

How can just one group change the perceptions of a profession and, ultimately, society in general? The legacy of the RSG is that the more visible this minority within a minority becomes, the easier it becomes for other GBLT people with disabilities to do the same.

This project to start the RSG was not something I set out to do. Rather, the idea to do so came to me, and I believe for a reason. I was in a good place to listen and respond to some of the subtle cues that were surfacing from around Connecticut.

Connecticut has a history of being more supportive of the sexual minority community than other places in the country (Connecticut Women's Education and Legal Fund [CWELF], 1995). It was the second state to repeal the sodomy laws in 1969, which criminalized homosexuality, and the third state in 1991 to offer civil rights protections for gay people (CWELF, 1995). Connecticut has a vibrant gay culture with businesses, institutions, and a visibility that is needed to encourage and support others in their desire to live an openly gay life.

As a long-term community activist and a human service professional, my office must have appeared to be a safe place to seek answers about GLBT people with intellectual disabilities. In addition, as the founder of the New Haven Gay & Lesbian Community Center, the process to create the Center was a public effort that frequently identified my employer and me in newspaper articles and television spotlights. Over a 2-year period, I logged more than a dozen statewide phone calls from staff desperately attempting to respond to the sexual orientation needs of their clients that, through neglect, had become a crisis. After receiving a particularly upsetting phone call, an idea materialized, and I implemented a plan of action. The action plan was to sponsor a focus group of progressive human service professionals who knew GBLT people with an intellectual or developmental disability or mental retardation willing to attend a support group meeting. Following several planning meetings over the next 6 months, consumers from throughout Connecticut were invited to what would quickly become the RSG.

I wanted to use the letterhead of my agency—a respected name in Connecticut—for a statewide announcement of the proposed group. The early support was necessary to counter any anticipated opposition.

Over the following 5 months, a series of planning meetings were held to gain support from agencies and staff, establish guidelines for participation and discussions, and begin educating the profession. Sexuality issues for people with intellectual or developmental disabilities or mental retardation are still considered, at best, an off-limits topic (Abbott & Howarth, 2003; Kempton, 1998). Not only were we faced with educating staff to acknowledge that clients can have a sexual orientation different from a heterosexual one, but also we had to educate them that clients are entitled to opportunities for privacy, intimacy, and sexual expression.

While the RSG has had a tremendous impact on the members, and hopefully within the profession, the activities of the group have changed little since the first meeting at the New Haven Gay & Lesbian Community Center in September 1998. The group has remained consistent both in size and topics of discussion. A core group of 10 to 20 members regularly attends group meetings, but over the years, more than 50 members have connected from around the state. Without question, the early State of Connecticut Department of Mental Retardation (DMR) support helped provide cover for those clients and staff interested in attending, and it also helped to silence any institutional homophobia that would inevitably have been directed at the group. While overt opposition to the group has been rare, there have been several instances when professional staff have either questioned the need for the group or stated that a program participant was merely confused. From the start, the RSG has been deliberate in broadcasting its message to the profession and the general community, which has certainly contributed to its success. If nothing else, the RSG has opened a dialogue to allow members, staff, and the general community to feel less inhibited by the subject.

THE GROUP AT HOME

The RSG has evolved into a support group for GLBT people with intellectual or developmental disabilities or mental retardation and others beginning to question their sexual orientation. All major components of the modern gay movement are represented in the group.

The RSG neither encourages or discourages developing relationships between members, but just like any other social or support group, members are able to develop friendships outside of the meetings. As members become more comfortable with one another over time, they have begun friendships with one another outside of the group.

The group meets monthly, on the second Monday of the month and always at the New Haven Gay & Lesbian Community Center. There are several reasons to meet at a gay center. As a focal point for gay life in Southern Connecticut, the Center hosts dozens of social and support groups, publishes a newsletter, has a web site, and produces many events during the year.

The Center offers RSG members an opportunity to soak up the surroundings by osmosis. For some, the time spent in the Center is their only gay experience, so it is not an insignificant detail. The Center is a clearinghouse for gay literature and periodicals and has a bulletin board for community postings. It is also home to many other groups and activities, which members are free to access on their own and indeed do. Through the RSG, the Center is more user-friendly, especially since the members have developed their own friends and a new reason to be in the space.

Many of the people that come to the RSG share similar characteristics surrounding their sexuality. Aware and socially alone in their sexual orientation, they can hold conflicting feelings about what they feel inside and how best to display those feelings within society and their personal support network. They are usually dependent on others for much of their daily living requirements, and if support staff and guardian family members have an anti-gay bias, RSG members may intuitively understand that a safe plan of action is to squelch the desire, or in other words, remain "in the closet." Many people who want to enjoy a shared sexual experience, and not just those with intellectual or developmental disabilities, may feel that the only outlets that they have are opportunistic encounters in such clandestine locations as public restrooms and parks (Blumenfeld, 1992). While staying "in the closet" may avoid confrontations with unsympathetic staff or family members, the unacknowledged desire can manifest not only in creating invisible personalities and greater dependency, but also in sneaky behaviors that leave the person open to assault, criminal actions, sexually transmitted diseases, and emotional turmoil.

After several years and dozens of members coming to the meetings, there are several personality traits that have surfaced. It became apparent that, although someone may identify as GLBT, it does not necessarily mean that he or she has acted on those desires. The individual may be able to articulate his or her feelings, but that does not indicate he or she has had gay experiences. A person can be gay without acting on the feelings, just as someone else can be heterosexual without becoming sexually involved with another person. Being gay reveals more about how a person feels inside than about their actions.

The RSG is an appropriate forum for members to connect with others to enjoy a shared gay experience. While some members may have never acted on their desires, the support group meetings and scheduled events serve an important function to bring people together into a gay space where they can at least participate in the community. The interaction serves to validate their feelings, build self-esteem, and counter some of the negative messages they may hold surrounding their sexual orientation. It is truly amazing to observe the initial reaction when someone new walks into the Center and realizes a sense of relief to have found a home. While not everyone will connect with a partner, participating in a community activity and sharing interactions with others who feel the same way is a part of the human experience everyone is entitled to enjoy.

WHAT IS TALKED ABOUT

If we as a profession believe that people with intellectual or developmental disabilities or mental retardation are entitled to make vocational, social, and residential choices, we should also respect their decisions for sexually intimate relationships. The RSG reveals that a person with an intellectual disability does have the intellectual capacity to decipher the intricacies of sexual orientation.

The members who attend the RSG are all able to articulate their feelings and demonstrate that they understand what it means to be part of the sexual minority community. The members come to the group with their own set of concerns, but they report an overwhelming sense of shared isolation and loneliness. At the very least, participation in the RSG gives members the opportunity to know other people with similar feelings.

Romance is a universal language that creates a normalizing effect for people with disabilities. While the RSG is not a dating service, companionship and the search for a partner is the primary issue discussed during meetings.

The desire for intimate relationships is articulated by every member of the RSG, but for people with intellectual disabilities, courtship is a process filled with complications and hurdles. While dating can be difficult for people without disabilities, the process can become insurmountable for those who have to accommodate to the additional demands of supervising staff dedicated to rules and routines. Too often, staff can maintain a posture of deliberate indifference toward such desires, which can manifest in other unproductive behaviors such as opportunistic sexual encounters in public facilities that can leave the person open to legal and safety risks.

People with intellectual disabilities are generally not encouraged to experiment with intimacy. While person-centered planning deals with many vocational and residential concerns, it can benignly neglect dating, relationships, and the desire for companionship. Sexuality, if discussed at all, is relegated to consultants who are specifically called when problems arise, such as someone acting inappropriately in public or displaying obsessive behavior toward staff or nondisabled associates.

The topics of conversations at the RSG meetings vary from mundane to personal to explicit perceptions and events. As with any other group, the conversation meanders as the focus goes around the room, but the members are always free to speak without the obligation of first censoring their gay perspective. Some members share stories about their work or recent community outings. Others like to discuss current events relating to gay issues. Every year, the group is invited to speak at several conferences where they have a chance to tell their stories and answer questions from the audience. The upcoming or previous RSG presentation experiences are a popular topic for discussion at monthly meetings. However, the topics most discussed during the meetings are the pursuit of relationships and how life in quasi-institutional group home settings restrict the members' opportunities to date and secure a partner. For 90 minutes once a month, members can feel the liberation, be nurtured by the environment, connect with others like them, and gather literature for home to carry them through another month.

SUCCESSES

The rainbow is a symbol of gay pride and solidarity (Marcus, 1993). In keeping with the symbol, the members named the group on the second meeting to declare their pride as gay people and their solidarity with the gay community.

Among the first of its kind in the nation, the RSG has been deliberately public with its message that some people with intellectual or developmental disabilities or mental retardation are gay. The RSG has garnered significant media coverage and serves as a clearinghouse for countless calls from around the country. Among many news stories, the RSG was featured in a national Associated Press article that appeared in several Connecticut Sunday newspapers including the *New Haven Register* (Greenberg, 1999) and a November 2000 national television broadcast on PBS stations (Karslake, 2000). Just by continuing to meet, the RSG is able to counter the stigma associated with mental retardation and sexual orientation.

The RSG is generating real change, literally one person at a time. Many members have no experiences in their life that delineates their "gayness," and yet they know they have feelings of same-sex attraction. The RSG provides an opportunity to at least have a shared experience where they can meet other people and learn about the gay community. By participating in the group, they can develop new friendships, attempt to arrange dates, and increase their chance of finding a partner. They can learn about appropriate ways to meet others, hear messages about safe sex, and feel empowered to advocate for their own intimacy needs.

Many members in the RSG have had success forming relationships with each other. For example, two lesbian members exchanged e-mail addresses following their first meeting together in February 2001, and by March they had declared the start of a relationship. Later that year, in November, they moved into their own apartment, supported by DMR, as an openly lesbian couple. The journey to assist them in their relationship was not without problems, but the same can happen in any relationship.

Other significant outcomes with the group involve several of the male members and their desire for dating and relationships. From the start, some of the male members dated one another. In retrospect, securing a partner seemed secondary to the activity of dating. It seemed they were more eager to date rather than actually obtain a boyfriend. It was when they were on the cusp of establishing a long-term commitment that problems emerged and there was wanderlust for unattainable staff and acquaintances.

Similarly, a transgender member who cross-dresses had endured tremendously difficult periods before finally finding support for his dream, which is to spend much of his leisure time cross-dressing. He had been threatened with blackmail, humiliated, manipulated, condemned, proselytized, and ignored, all for what seemed natural to him. Here is a man who works, earns his own money, maintains an apartment, and is his own legal guardian, and yet his time and desires were not his own. The RSG was a quiet force to assist him in connecting with support staff who wanted only to listen to him and not try to force him to conform to someone else's expectations.

What has also surfaced as RSG members speak at conferences around the country is that the profession has done little to address the desire of all people with intellectual disabilities to have opportunities for intimacy. The RSG is doing more than just advocating for sexual minority people with cognitive impairments. It has become a catalyst to begin discussing sexuality in general for the heterosexual majority. Sexuality is the elephant in the room given the reliance on government funding and the public perception of sexuality as a politically loaded term (Hingsburger, 1991). While many direct care support staff either avoid the topic or are moralistic about sexuality, there is an underlying feeling of frustration and powerlessness to be able to assist the people they serve with such an important and deeply private aspect of life (Monat-Haller, 1992). It is surprising that RSG, a group that represents a minority of people with intellectual or developmental disabilities or mental retardation, is actually assisting the rest of the community in bringing about a discussion of the rights of all individuals to experience sexual expression. For example, during one of the self-determination conferences, a state worker was incredulous when he asked, "How can you talk about homosexuality when we can't talk about any kind of sexuality?" Part of the success of the group can be attributed to a deliberate effort to broadcast a message that sexual orientation and gender identity variations are part of the human experience that deserve to be celebrated. Additionally, because of the uniqueness of the group, several heterosexually identified people with intellectual or developmental disabilities or mental retardation have either attended or have become members so as to have a forum to discuss sexual expression in a supportive environment.

The RSG is building a framework for what is surely to come later. Its success is in the ability of its members to live open and honest lives. Sexuality is a natural component of being an adult, and to deny someone access to his or her feelings renders the person invisible. Ultimately, the power of the RSG is in its self-advocacy and declaration of purpose.

OVERCOMING ADVERSITY

The RSG is such a tremendous source of strength for its members, and an educational resource for the profession, that it seems counterproductive to discuss any of the obstacles to its success. However, the issues raised here serve as a reminder that triumphs rise from adversity.

As the founder and a facilitator of the RSG, my name serves as a flash point for family members and staff uncomfortable with GLBT issues, but also for members and other clients who are grappling with their own sexual orientation. The RSG is a member-driven group where we talk about whatever is on the members' minds, and we try to respond if not with cohesion, then with support. During a particularly difficult period in the group, when we were waiting for a national television feature to air on public broadcasting stations, several family members and staff had a typical reaction to our very public "outing." Homosexuality continues to be viewed as taboo, although this viewpoint is rapidly changing to be considered as part of the human condition. Very often, when gay people come out of the closet, family members and friends can have the exact opposite reaction and go into the closet! For some people, disclosure, even of association with homosexuality, can be laden with embarrassment and guilt (Bernstein, 1995).

Some of the members that attend the RSG are their own legal guardians, in which they have the legal right to make their own decisions. Still, that does not preclude concerned family members from getting involved in their decisions.

The RSG is a controversial group because it involves the subject of sexuality in the disabilities community, which is often a taboo subject. A family member of an RSG member was aware that his adult child was attending the group, but he took umbrage at some of the publicity surrounding the television feature partly because his child was prominently featured.

"If you were truly interested in helping them, you would do it quietly and not celebrate [homosexuality]," said the parent, suggesting that I coerced the members to appear on television.

My response was that I was a human service professional obligated to listen to the messages of my clients. Without publicity in the general community to help normalize the subject, the group was at risk of losing its momentum. My response was, "The best way to make life better for the members is to celebrate who they are."

It is difficult to take an in-between stance when it comes to celebrating who you are (Savin-Williams, 2001). Can you be a little bit gay? How do you make a quiet public announcement about a unique group in a local community? A public message is just that—public—and since there is so much anxiety surrounding the sexuality of people with intellectual or developmental disabilities or mental retardation, there are many people who feel that a public dialogue on the subject should be introduced more slowly, if at all.

The courageous person during this episode was the RSG member. At the next meeting, following the exchange with the parent, the member said to another member who was also going through a similar experience with family members, "Stick up for your rights. I did."

It is estimated that up to 3% of the population experiences mental retardation, or 8.4 million people in the United States (The Arc, 2004). If only a small number of those Americans are members of the GLBT community, there is still much work to do to provide support in the human service profession. Even if the numbers are only a fraction at 1% or 2%, service providers still need to put aside their personal biases toward sexuality and sexual orientation to assist the people they serve. So the question becomes, how can we best reach those people about the message of the RSG?

There is a dilemma in trying to broadcast the message of a controversial subject. If the message is too blatant, it offends many conservative stakeholders, but if it is too vague, the message is easily ignored or fails to generate interest. Trying to find the right balance in disseminating information on the RSG has been a source of many of the battles encountered. As a member-driven group, the members have been united in their effort to be public with the message in the media, within the state provider network, and within other self-advocacy groups. As evidence that the tactic has been successful, several other RSG groups around the country have formed or are in the process of forming, and the Connecticut group continues to be invited to conferences to share their stories of coming out as openly GLBT people who happen to experience intellectual or developmental disabilities or mental retardation. As a unique group, part of the strategy in validating the RSG has been to entrench the group in institutional and professional structures. While media has been one of the legs of support, forging formal and informal links with human service and gay community organizations has also contributed to maintaining a viable group. Creating a network of contacts has increased the likelihood that the group will be considered for referrals, welcomed at gay events, and invited to professional conferences. The approach, once again, creates a more visible group, which can challenge the comfort level of even the staunchest supporter.

One of the more proactive administrators at an agency that has consistently demonstrated their support for the RSG and for acknowledging the sexuality of their clients was faced with such a scenario. In preparation for an awards ceremony, several individuals and organizations were nominated for their support of the RSG. The award was the Jane Addams Award (Jane Addams is the founder of the social work movement) for institutional courage from the Connecticut Coalition for LGBT Civil Rights—a prestigious gay community organization dedicated to civil rights. The group is modeled after other civil rights organizations, such as the NAACP and the ADL.

After submitting a lengthy application and sharing copies with key players, the administrator called to say that the nomination had breached a confidence and had to be immediately rescinded. The primary concerns were that the town where they are located is a working class community where gay issues are not part of the local dialogue. The board of directors for the agency was also unaware of the quiet support that had been offered by the administrator.

During a follow-up meeting in which we both had a more relaxed opportunity to explain our actions, the crux of the dilemma in advancing the goals of the RSG was revealed. A new organization needs to generate awareness and credentials as it attempts to build a network. For the administrator, the reaction exemplified the internalized homophobia we all must overcome to fully embrace the message of the RSG.

"Would you have had the same reaction if you were nominated for a Jane Addams Award from the NAACP? Would you have declined to accept a Jane Addams Award from the ADL?" I asked, without expecting or receiving a reply.

Similarly, at a statewide conference on intellectual or developmental disabilities and mental retardation where the RSG was invited to present a seminar, a description of the RSG was sent beforehand for publication in a conference guide. The description had been edited, without permission or notification, which created great confusion once the presentation began for some attendees who expected something else.

The submitted description was as follows:

> The RSG provides a safe space for discussion and fellowship among people with developmental disabilities who are Gay, Lesbian, Bisexual, and Transgender. This emerging issue, along with sexuality and relationships, will be discussed.

The edited description, however, appeared as such:

> The RSG provides a safe space for discussion and fellowship among people with developmental disabilities who have alternative lifestyles. This emerging issue, along with sexuality and relationships, will be discussed.

Using words to define one's own life and describe components of one's personality is an empowering exercise for people who continue to

be treated as if they are invisible. It was ironic that the planners of a conference on self-determination would ignore their own mission and
attempt to sanitize the message after accepting a presentation in the
hope that it would not offend some of the more conservative attendees.
What occurred in the process was that the presenters, and the very attendees the seminar was designed to reach, were the ones who were deeply
offended.

I believe that the most powerful tool the gay community can use to
effect change is also a personal one—it is to simply come out, to tell
their stories of growing up, and describe their feelings. The closet is a
prison and has been effectively used against gay people and for anyone
that considers his or her sexuality a source of shame (Bernstein, 1995).
The resistance to come out is so powerful that many are unable to challenge what has typically been a lifelong assault. It is because of the injus-
tices I see and experience everyday as an openly gay man, that I do not
want anyone else who is gay, lesbian, bisexual, or transgender to be told
that they are anything less than unique and valued and can have a life
filled with great potential.

CONCLUSION

What I have most learned in this journey to provide a safe place within
the human service profession and the gay community, is the power of
the human spirit. The members who come to the RSG have endured
some of the most inhumane conditions and difficult circumstances and
yet, their generosity and optimism shines at every meeting. Their insight
into complex relationships reads as sophisticated beyond expectations.
The desire to build a sense of community is real as they respond to their
own inner voices.

The RSG stands ready to serve as a model throughout the profession for other states and regions to create similar support groups for
their clients. Already, the RSG has provided inspiration for other
regions, in Massachusetts, Minnesota, and Vermont, as more human
service staff recognizes the diversity within the disabilities community.
The best course of action for the RSG is to simply continue to do what
it has done successfully since September of 1998—to provide a safe and
inviting environment for GLBT people with intellectual or developmental disabilities or mental retardation.

During a recent conversation, a key administrator at a member's
agency called to voice a concern that a frequent topic at the monthly
meetings was encouraging unrealistic expectations for the client. Since

the client lives in an intensively supervised residential setting, it would be virtually impossible to allow any opportunities for intimacy or a close personal relationship.

"I can respect your position and will try to be more sensitive to your concerns," I replied, trying to remain cognizant that the comment came from an ally not an adversary, and then added a caveat. "Having quality of life is more than just having a full belly and a warm place to sleep. Aren't we all looking for relationships and the opportunity to share our life with a partner?"

So what if a person lives under constant supervision? Is it not our obligation, as human service professionals, to ensure that people we support with disabilities have the same opportunities to realize their dreams in life? Just as heterosexuals do not have a monopoly on sexuality, the potential for having a relationship is not limited to intellectual privilege—it is part of what makes us human. What the RSG has accomplished and will hopefully continue to illuminate is the understanding that people with intellectual or developmental disabilities and mental retardation are entitled to a whole life experience, including discovering and enjoying their sexuality.

REFERENCES

Abbott, D., & Howarth, J. (February, 2003). A secret love, a hidden life. *Learning Disability Practice, 6*(1), 14–17.

Bernstein, R.A. (1995). *Straight parents, gay children: Keeping families together.* New York: Thunder's Mouth Press.

Blumenfeld, W.J. (1992). *Homophobia: How we all pay the price.* Boston: Beacon Press.

Connecticut Women's Education and Legal Fund. (1995). *The legal rights of lesbians and gay men in Connecticut* (3rd ed.) [Brochure]. Hartford, CT: Author.

Duberman, M. (1993). *Stonewall.* New York: Penguin.

Gay & Lesbian Alliance Against Defamation. (2001). *Lesbian, gay, bisexual & transgender media reference guide.* [Brochure]. New York: Author.

Greenberg, B. (1999, December 19). For the disabled, sexuality is real. *New Haven Register,* pp. B1, B4.

Hingsburger, D. (1991). *I contact: Sexuality and people with developmental disabilities.* Mountville, PA: VIDA Publishing.

Kempton, W. (1998). *Sex education for persons with disabilities that hinder learning: A teacher's guide.* Santa Barbara, CA: James Stanfield Company.

Karslake, D. (Producer). (2000, November). Episode 1002 [Television series episode]. *In the life television.* Arlington, VA: Public Broadcasting Service.

Marcus, E. (1993). *Is it a choice: Answers to 300 of the most frequently asked questions about gays and lesbians.* New York: HarperCollins.

Monat-Haller, R.K. (1992). *Understanding & expressing sexuality: Responsible choices for individuals with developmental disabilities.* Baltimore: Paul H. Brookes Publishing Co.

Savin-Williams, R.C. (2001). *Mom, Dad. I'm gay: How families negotiate coming out.* Washington, DC: American Psychological Association.

The Arc. (2004). *Introduction to mental retardation.* Retrieved October 5, 2005, from http://www.thearc.org/faqs/mrqa.doc

III

Risk Management Related to Sexual Choices

9

Consent to Sexual Activity

Legal and Clinical Considerations

Ruth Luckasson and Leslie Walker-Hirsch

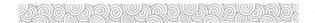

This chapter explores the legal and clinical issues around consent to sexual activity when one or both parties have an intellectual disability. First, we examine the purposes of laws generally and analyze what roles laws play in a society. Then, we analyze various unique aspects of sexual activity that present special challenges to the law. Next, we explore the interaction of sexuality and law and the range of goals that laws might have in the sexuality arena. We go on to review the application to individuals of laws affecting sexuality through typical civil laws and criminal laws of a state. Finally, we summarize the consent and competency issues central to the laws on sexuality and disability, describe how the clinical considerations are related to legal considerations, and recommend considerations for professionals who are asked to contribute information and opinion to evaluations of an individual's consent for sexual activity.

ROLES OF LAW IN SOCIETY

Most people probably live the sexual aspects of their lives without giving much thought to the law. After all, we might think, why should something so private and individual, so personal between intimate partners, require the involvement of law? But the law plays an important part in the societal regulation of sexuality. Let's examine why that might be.

What is the role of law in a society? Law, especially in a participatory democracy, strives to protect citizens from dangers such as aggression from other people or unconstitutional intrusions by the government. It also strives to enhance the well-being and liberties of its citizens. The important roles that the law plays in our society include helping to express a common vision, communicate widely held values, set standards of behavior, and create predictability, protection, and mechanisms for safe dispute resolution.

How does law express and formalize a society's widely held values and articulate a common vision for a community? American laws prohibit battery of another person and specify punishments for people who violate the criminal laws against battery (see, e.g., N.M. Stat. 1978 section 30-3-4 [1963] for definition of criminal battery). These laws help to institutionalize and formalize the high value our society places on the physical integrity and safety of each person. Laws also set standards and expectations for individual behavior. Publicizing and enforcing laws against battery, for example, sends the message to all individuals in the society that the standard of behavior is that no one is allowed to touch another person unless they have the person's permission or agreement.

The rule of law also enhances everyday predictability about many aspects of community life for citizens. It communicates to people what they can expect in their society and helps provide order. Without laws, individuals are subject to societal disorder and unpredictability, which undermine the social contract and cause the threads of a society to unravel. In addition, laws can help protect vulnerable groups from the unfettered power of stronger groups, and laws are essential to the organization of safe dispute resolution mechanisms. If individuals do not have access to safe means such as legal prosecutions and lawsuits to resolve the inevitable disputes that arise between people, they would likely resort to disorderly and unsafe means such as physical aggression to solve their disputes, and society would suffer (Rawls, 1971).

LEGAL REGULATION OF SEXUALITY

Many sexuality-related behaviors are subject to legal regulation. Because the law attempts to represent the beliefs at a particular time for the broadest common group of people, it does not always reflect the most current beliefs or quickly accommodate to societal changes and unique and unexpected circumstances of particular individuals. As a result, individuals sometimes object to the law's attempt to regulate sexual activities that they have an interest in but that are different from the current legal interpretation of permissible sexual activity. Mechanisms for altering the law are anticipated within the law, but making changes in the law is often cumbersome and slow.

States often have legal restrictions on the age of consent for certain activities, the number and gender of marital partners a person may have at a given time (e.g., laws prohibiting polygamy, laws prohibiting certain gay, lesbian, bisexual, transgender activities), and the types of sexual intercourse. Why do some sexuality-related behaviors receive this legal attention? There are a number of likely reasons for this attention. Some sexual activities can encroach upon or intrude into the personal integrity of others. Some activities have potential risks and can lead to irreversible and undesirable consequences. Consider, for example, that forms of sexual expression, such as sexual intercourse, are potentially very powerful—emotionally, physically, and socially—for the participating individuals. And sometimes the sexual expression also involves significant power imbalances between the individuals, which can lead to victimization. In addition, many expressions of sexuality are quite personal, private, and intimate, and go to the core of a person's individual identity. Thus, individuals have strong feelings about intrusions to their identity and have strong feelings about how they are treated sexually by others. Moreover, the individuality and personal autonomy of every person are extremely highly valued in our society. Despite the fact that individual freedom is vitally important, the law is not always able to resolve the tension between protecting citizens and assuring their maximum personal liberty. The law must constantly attempt to balance possible oppression against possible benefit, within the framework of the Constitution. Some sexual activities carry high risk of unintended consequences, such as pregnancy or disease; some of these consequences are undesirable and/or irreversible. Thus, it becomes clear that a society would want to have rules and send clear messages about sexual activity in order to establish certain behavioral expectations in the society to reduce disruption and to maintain the orderliness of essential institutions.

The law seeks to regulate sexual activities that involve potential power imbalances, uncontrolled physical consequences, potential risks to safety and health, and threats to orderly social interactions and property ownership. Therefore, not every sexual activity is regulated by the law. Stavis and Walker-Hirsch (1999) suggested three levels of sexual activity, which correspond to three levels of legal scrutiny (see Table 9.1). The level of legal scrutiny is generally based on the risk, intrusiveness, and irreversibility of the activity (American Association on Mental Retardation, 1977). Consider the three levels.

Table 9.1.   Levels of monitoring consent

Level of legal scrutiny	Level of risk, intrusiveness, irreversibility	Examples of activities
Minimal monitoring	Low risk, low intrusiveness, usually reversible consequences	Friendship; holding hands; dancing; adult print, electronic, and media material; masturbation or other self-stimulatory sexual behavior
Moderate monitoring to assure mutual agreement	Limited risk, moderate intrusiveness, moderate risk of irreversible consequences	Mutually agreed-upon erotic activities, such as intimate conversation, prolonged kissing, petting, cooperative sex play
Formal monitoring and assurance of adequate consent, especially for identified vulnerable individuals	High risk, high intrusiveness, high risk of reversible or irreversible and undesirable consequences	Sexual activities involving genital fluid exchange, such as vaginal, anal, and oral intercourse

From Stavis, P.F., & Walker-Hirsch, L. (1999). Consent to sexual activity. In R.D. Dinerstein, S.S. Herr, & J.L. O'Sullivan (Eds.), *A guide to consent* (pp. 57–67). Washington, DC: American Association on Mental Retardation. Adapted with permission.

Legal regulation of sexual activity worldwide is also influenced by the culture, form of government, social structure, and status of the parties. For example, until the late 1970s, it was legally impossible in most states in the United States for a husband to be criminally prosecuted for rape of his wife because the status of a wife was to be owned and controlled by the husband (Russel, 1990). In some cultures, where women do not have status and men hold all of the power, consent to intercourse or absence of consent are irrelevant—there remain exemptions from criminal penalties for men who, for example, subsequently marry their kidnapped, raped, or assaulted victim (Equality Now, 2004). Similarly, until individuals with disabilities were recognized as autonomous human beings having rights, they were assumed to be permanent children or lower beings in need of lifelong protection and external control. They were believed to be either asexual or oversexed, or always incapable of consenting to any sexual activity.

Now the human rights status of all people with disabilities is recognized (see, e.g., Herr, Gostin, & Koh, 2003; Quinn & Degener, 2002; United Nations General Assembly, 2001). It is clear that education about sexuality, pursuit of personal choices, and achieving adult status and relationships are critical to the life satisfaction of many adults with intellectual disabilities. But challenges remain in balancing their rights to adult status, including decisions about sexual activities, with possible lack of consent, vulnerability to power imbalances, aggressive behavior from or toward others, health risks, and unwanted pregnancies. Cognitive limitations can cause an individual to be more vulnerable in situations requiring problem solving, judgment, and communication—which is why people need supports. In the sexuality area, these supports may include evaluation, specialized education, increased supervision, supported or joint decision making, counseling, and personal futures planning, to name a few.

The legal regulation of sexual activities is almost exclusively within the state law arena. Therefore, it is critical for individuals with intellectual disabilities, their families, and support professionals to know about the relevant laws in their states. The laws are found in both the civil law and the criminal law, depending on the issue.

COMMON CIVIL LAW REGULATION OF SEXUAL ACTIVITIES

In the civil law arena, it is important to know your state's relevant laws concerning guardianship, sterilization, abuse reporting, tort liability and malpractice, professional licensing, research, and privacy.

One of the most important civil law areas for people with cognitive disabilities is the state's guardianship law. If an individual has a legal guardian, it is critical to understand what type of guardianship has been imposed, what the powers of the guardian are, whether the guardian can control where the person lives and who he or she can see, and whether the guardian has the power to authorize (or prevent) access to critical decisions involving sexuality, such as choice of friends, involvement in sexuality education, selection of birth control, or even surgical sterilization. However, it is important to note that while a guardian may in some cases withhold critical choices about sexual matters from a person in whose interest they act as a guardian, they may *not* consent for a person, as a surrogate consent agent, if the person does not have the present capacity to consent for him- or herself.

It is also important to check the state's law on involuntary surgical sterilization, if applicable. Generally, only a court can authorize involuntary sterilization, even then, it can do so only under significant protections (see, e.g., In re Hayes, 1980). States differ, however, on the precise nature of the legal protections.

Civil abuse law should also be consulted. States require the reporting of suspected abuse of children and vulnerable adults. It is important to know what is defined as abuse in your state, who has a duty to report, and how and to whom one must report. The health laws for reporting communicable diseases such as sexually transmitted diseases (STDs) should also be consulted.

Knowledge of the state's law on tort liability for civil wrongs such as malpractice actions against professionals and agencies is also important. The legal elements of a malpractice claim are duty, breach of duty, damages, and causation (see Chapter 10). It is essential that sexuality professionals use best practices, which includes professional ethics, professional standards, research-based knowledge, and appropriate clinical judgment (Schalock & Luckasson, 2005). Professionals should appropriately document their actions. But justice also depends on increasing public education concerning incorrect stereotypes about people with intellectual disabilities and sexuality, including misinformation held by judges and juries.

Many professional licensing statutes also contain relevant provisions. Professionals who have been found to have violated certain prohibitions concerning sexual activities may find their professional licenses revoked. For example, in New Mexico, a physical therapist who engages in or solicits a sexual relationship with a patient, whether consensual or not, is subject to disciplinary action, including revocation of his/her professional license (N.M. Stat. 1978 section 61-12D-13 [1997]).

It is also important to investigate relevant research and privacy laws. Consent is required before evaluating an individual, in order to protect privacy, and also for an individual's participation in a research study.

COMMON CRIMINAL LAW REGULATION OF SEXUAL ACTIVITIES

The state's definition of consent forms the crux of almost all of the criminal law issues regarding intellectual disability and sexuality. As a general matter, the definition will include some formulation of the three elements of consent: capacity, information, and voluntariness (Dinerstein, Herr, & O'Sullivan, 1999). It is important to become familiar with your state's definition because the definitions vary in the terms used and other essential matters, such as whether an evaluation is necessary and who may conduct it.

State laws prohibiting sexual intercourse without consent vary considerably. Generally, the laws on consent require finding some combination of the following: understanding the nature of the sexual conduct, understanding of and ability to exercise the right to refuse the activity, understanding possible risks and consequences, and appreciation of moral dimensions and societal taboos. State law, however, can never precisely quantify the required amounts of capacity, information, and voluntariness. Thus, evaluations must incorporate the clinical judgment of the evaluators and reflect the individually determined personal skills, goals, and values of the person being evaluated.

Similarly, the state will have criminal battery laws, criminal abuse laws, and perhaps penalty enhancements depending on the vulnerable status of the victim.

According to the American Association on Mental Retardation (AAMR; Dinerstein, Herr, & O'Sullivan, 1999), in order for a person to be able to provide legally adequate consent, he or she must be able to demonstrate three broad elements:

- Capacity: Meeting a minimum age requirement as well as being able to demonstrate relevant personal decision making, functional understanding, and meaningful communication
- Information: Receiving knowledge that is adequate in both quality and quantity
- Voluntariness: Exercising free and uncoerced choice

Some states have an additional requirement that the person demonstrate their understanding of the social and moral implications of their acts.

Most of the time, we presume that an adult automatically has the ability to give consent. There are times, however, when even adults do not have that capacity, not only when we are under the influence of alcohol or drugs, which render us unable to reason, or when we undergo anesthesia and are unconscious, which renders us temporarily unable to give consent not only to sexual activity, but also to many other important activities, such as entering into contracts. Under these circumstances, the loss of ability is temporary or planned for until our ability to give or withhold consent is restored. We are not questioned or evaluated about our capacity but the presumption of capacity is made. However, when there are factors or circumstances that cause doubt about whether an individual can consent or not, further investigation may be needed. Consent of adults who have been determined to have intellectual disabilities cannot always be presumed. Further investigation may be required to determine if the disability interferes with the person's ability to give consent. Determining clinically if a person can give consent by evaluating the factors needed is the safeguard against incorrectly assuming consent when it may not exist. And, conversely, presuming lack of consent simply because a person has an intellectual disability may deprive the person of rights to which he or she is entitled. If you help a person who is not consenting to access non-consensual sex, then YOU may be accused of a serious crime. What does this mean?

The first element for consent is capacity. A person can be evaluated on his or her capacity by determining the person's age, general knowledge, and ability. It will be important to evaluate whether the person has learned or can be taught to make relevant decisions, whether he or she genuinely and functionally understands what is at issue, and whether he or she can meaningfully communicate his or her understanding and decisions.

The second element for consent is information or knowledge. A person can be evaluated to ascertain his or her level of information about the activity that he or she has interest in, and whether it is enough knowledge to provide a reasonable degree of safety. The person needs to be able to recognize that the acts of interest themselves are sexual in nature, and the person must be able to differentiate them from other acts that are not sexual. The person must know the risks and benefits of engaging in sexual activities. This factor of consent is usually met through successfully achieving the learning objectives of a comprehensive sexuality education program. Consider this: If a person is deprived of sex education in school or adult programs, how will that person meet this measure for consent?

The third element of consent is voluntariness. Does the person have the ability to reason about making choices in life? Does the person show that he or she can make choices about what to wear on a frigid day or choices about what to do when he or she is hungry or thirsty? A person who believes he or she is receiving commands from the TV and cannot distinguish those from auditory events that others can verify may not have adequate reasoning ability to make voluntary choices. There needs to be no element of coercion surrounding the decision for sexual contact. Indeed sexual abuse is sometimes defined as forcing, threatening, tricking, coaxing, or manipulating another person into unwanted sexual contact or into sexual contact to which the person does not have the capacity to consent. Michael Smull reported that he and other professionals favor that voluntariness be shown in an active way because people with intellectual disabilities are often overly compliant and acquiescent to the suggestions and demands of others, especially those of authority figures (personal communication, July 2005). Active voluntariness may be shown by actions such as preparing to have a sexual encounter or making a joint sexual decision with another person with the help of a counselor to guide and support the couple. Many would agree that active participation in a couples group would show lack of coercion if intention was made known during that time to other group members.

The sometimes specified fourth element of consent regarding the social and moral implications of a particular activity is the least well defined. The personal values of the individual and the overriding social milieu of a specific community at a specific point in time may not be in harmony or may be unknowable by a person with an intellectual disability. When sexual matters are not openly discussed within families or adult programs, the discussion of personal values regarding sexual activity and of family perceptions of "right and wrong" can "go underground" and be deliberately kept from family or other caregivers. As a result there will be no check on the veracity or adequacy of the information.

When consent is in question a professional may be called upon to gather information about these elements and report the findings to a decision-making team or committee. The professional may rely on pictorial supports or unique materials to ascertain this information. Or, perhaps readymade consent assessments, such as *Tool for Assessing Informed Sexual Consent Through an Evaluation of Responsible Sexual Behavior* (YAI, 2003) or *Sexuality Safety Skills and Support Needs Assessment Tool, Second Edition* (Ray Graham Association for People with Disabilities, 2005) will be adequate to address these concerns. When all three (or four, depending on the state law) of these elements for consent are met, in the opinion of the team or committee, the person is determined to be consenting under the current circumstance. But as we know, consent is not static, and circumstances change as well.

When a person is judged as NOT having adequate consent, what is the responsibility of the agency, team, or professional? The team should make every effort to advance the person toward becoming able to consent. This might mean additional education, improved social opportunity, practice in decision making, or environmental changes that redirect the person toward some lower risk activity that the person can manage right away.

Documentation that shows that the specified agency policy was followed and that best professional practice was adhered to should help protect the clinicians, the agency, and the person from assertions that their actions constituted breach of duty and caused harm to the individual.

When individuals with intellectual disabilities are involved in the criminal justice system, they are most often the victims of crimes (Luckasson, 1992; Petersilia, 2001). But individuals with intellectual disabilities might also be accused of committing a crime. Professionals must be prepared to consider situations in which the defendant might have an intellectual disability, situations in which the victim has an intellectual disability, or situations in which both defendant and alleged victim have intellectual disabilities. When the defendant has an intellectual disability, likely legal issues include *competence to confess, competence to stand trial,* and *competence to waive Constitutional rights*. When the victim has an intellectual disability, an additional likely legal issue is *competence to testify* (Conley, Luckasson, & Bouthilet, 1992; Ellis & Luckasson, 1985; Luckasson & Vance, 1995).

In summary, in the criminal law arena, it is important to know your state's relevant criminal laws concerning rape, battery, criminal sexual abuse, harassment, and any enhancement of penalty provisions that are related to the victim's disability. It is also important to be familiar with doctrines such as *competence to stand trial, competence to confess,* and *competence to waive Constitutional rights* that might be relevant if the defendant has an intellectual disability, and *competence to testify* which might be relevant if the alleged victim has an intellectual disability.

The authoritative analysis of legally adequate consent for individuals with intellectual disabilities is found in *A Guide to Consent* published by the AAMR (Dinerstein et al., 1999). This work must always be considered in the context of your state's law on consent.

CONSIDERATIONS FOR PROFESSIONALS WHO ARE ASKED TO CONTRIBUTE INFORMATION

When a professional is asked to contribute to an evaluation of whether an individual can consent to sexual activity, the professional must clarify several factors:

- What is the purpose of the evaluation?
- Who will make the decision about consent?
- What are the relevant state laws?
- What is the professional's role?

It may also be useful for the professional to indicate in the body of the report the limits of the professional's contribution. Leslie Walker-Hirsch, one of the authors of this chapter, often includes the following guiding statement in her clinical evaluations, "This report may be used *to assist* a Consent Evaluation Team/Committee to decide whether an individual meets the standards for consent. It does **not** represent a decision regarding informed or meaningful consent." Ideally, decisions regarding consent should be the result of properly documented team decision making that includes the individual who is being evaluated and people who are familiar with that individual's abilities, history, and desires for the future. The team members should attempt to reach a consensus about consent or about how to assist that individual to increase his or her ability and perhaps move toward meeting the standards for consent.

Stavis and Walker-Hirsch (1999) suggested professionals consider the following questions when asked to be a contributing member of a consent evaluation committee.

Consider whether the person:

1. Is an adult, as defined by state law

2. Demonstrates an awareness of person, time, place, and event

3. Possesses a basic knowledge of sexual activities

4. Possesses the skills to participate safely in sexual activities, that is, consider whether the person understands how and why to effectively use an appropriate method of birth control and whether the person chooses to do so

5. Understands the physical and legal responsibilities of pregnancy

6. Is aware of sexually transmittable diseases and how to avoid them

7. Demonstrates an awareness of legal implications concerning wrongful sexual behaviors (e.g., sexual assault, inappropriateness of sex with minors, exploitation)

8. Can identify when others' rights are infringed

9. Demonstrates that "no" from another person means to stop (i.e., understands that it is always inappropriate to have sex or engage in other activities with someone who says no or otherwise objects by words or actions)

10. Knows when sexual advances are appropriate as to time and place (e.g., different places and times may apply to dancing, touching, or sexual intercourse)

11. Does not allow his or her own disability to be exploited by a partner

12. Knows when both parties are agreeing to the same sexual activity

13. Does not exploit another person with lower functioning who might not be able to say no or defend him- or herself

14. Expresses understandable responses to life experiences (i.e., can accurately report events)

15. Can describe the decision-making process used to make the choice to engage in sexual activity

16. Demonstrates the ability to differentiate between truth, fantasy, and lies

17. Possesses a reasoning process that includes an expression of individual values

18. Can reasonably execute choices associated with a judgmental process

19. Is able to identify and recognize the feelings expressed by others, both verbally and nonverbally

20. Expresses emotions consistent with the actual or proposed sexual situation

21. Rejects unwanted advances or intrusions to protect oneself from sexual exploitation

22. Identifies and uses private rooms or areas for intimate behavior

23. Is able to call for help or report unwanted advances or abuse

24. Rejects high-risk or inappropriate sexual activity to meet needs that can be better met in ways that involve less risk, are more appropriate, or do not require consent (adapted from Stavis & Walker-Hirsch, 1999, pp. 63–64)

While the list is long, the purpose of the list is not to be a test for the person with the disability; rather, the list represents documentation of the factors that the professional has considered in the evaluation. The professional's documentation of information pertaining to the items on the list can contribute to the verification of professional practice.

The answers to these questions will not only summarize the current functional capacity of the individual but should also suggest environmental and programmatic modifications to support the person and move the person closer to meeting the standards necessary for participation in the desired activity.

The legal regulation of sexual activity is most relevant when the intrusion, risk, and irreversibility are highest. Most frequently, the legal issue is consent. As discussed previously, legally adequate consent requires three elements: capacity, information, and voluntariness. But consent can fluctuate—it is not a static one-time-for-all-activities decision. With maturation, learning, and experience, an individual may be able to gain the ability to consent. A dream of a richer life in the future that might include desired sexual activity can be a powerful motivator for a person to make the required effort for personal growth and achievement. The resulting optimism can contribute to mental health and personal satisfaction. But even if an individual never is able to provide legally adequate consent for sexual intercourse, he or she may be able to provide agreement to dance with a friend or hold hands on a date. The law should enhance the lives and liberty of individuals with intellectual disabilities while protecting those who are vulnerable from serious danger and assuring them of justice if harm occurs.

All individuals are unique, and each person's choices about sexuality reflect that uniqueness. Risk is an inherent part of all activities, including sexual activities. It is the role of professionals to evaluate a vulnerable person's ability to consent, but it is the person's role to make informed and deeply personal choices consistent with his or her own ability, culture, values, and the law. The law must be sufficiently flexible to respect not just a person's sexuality skills and limitations but also less tangible factors such as temperament, risk tolerance, aspirations, and the right to create one's own future. Sexuality clinicians must be sufficiently skilled to capture and contribute an accurate reflection of a person's abilities and dreams so that the law can support the best balance of protection from harm and enhancement of well-being and liberty.

REFERENCES

American Association of Mental Retardation. (1977). *Consent handbook.* Washington, DC: Author.

Conley, R., Luckasson, R., & Bouthilet, G. (Eds.) (1992). *The criminal justice system and mental retardation: Defendants and victims.* Baltimore: Paul H. Brookes Publishing Co.

Dinerstein, R.D., Herr, S.S., & O'Sullivan, J.L. (1999). *A guide to consent.* Washington, DC: American Association on Mental Retardation.

Ellis, J.W., & Luckasson, R. (1985). Mentally retarded criminal defendants. *George Washington Law Review, 53,* 414–494.

Equality Now. (2004). *Words and deeds: Holding governments accountable in the Beijing + 10 review process.* Retrieved November 6, 2005, from http://www.equalitynow.org/english/wan/beijing10/beijing10_en.pdf

Herr, S.S., Gostin, L.O., & Koh, H.H. (2003). *The human rights of persons with intellectual disabilities: Different but equal.* New York: Oxford.

In re Hayes, 608 P. 2d 635 (Wash. 1980).

Luckasson, R. (1992). People with mental retardation as victims of crime. In R. Conley, R. Luckasson, & G. Bouthilet (Eds.), *The criminal justice system and mental retardation: Defendants and victims* (pp. 209–220). Baltimore: Paul H. Brookes Publishing Co.

Luckasson, R., & Vance, E. (Eds.) (1995). *Defendants, victims, and witnesses with mental retardation: An instructional guide for judges and judicial educators.* Reno, NV: The National Judicial College.

N.M. Stat. 1978 section 30-3-4 (1963).

N.M. Stat. 1978 section 61-12D-13 (1997).

Petersilia, J. R. (2001). Crime victims with developmental disabilities: A review essay. *Criminal Justice and Behavior, 28*(6), 655–694.

Quinn, G., & Degener, T. (2002). *Human rights and disability: The current use and future potential of United Nations human rights instruments in the context of disability.* New York and Geneva: Author.

Rawls, J. (1971). *A theory of justice.* Cambridge, MA: Belknap Press of Harvard.

Ray Graham Association for People with Disabilities. (2005). *Sexuality safety skills and support needs assessment tool* (2nd. ed.). Downer's Grove, IL: Ray Graham Association.

Russel, E.H. (1990). *Rape in marriage: Expanded and revised edition with a new introduction.* Bloomington: Indiana University Press.

Schalock, R.L., & Luckasson, R. (2005). *Clinical judgment.* Washington, DC: American Association on Mental Retardation.

Stavis, P.F., & Walker-Hirsch, L. (1999). Consent to sexual activity. In R.D. Dinerstein, S.S. Herr, & J.L. O'Sullivan (Eds.), *A guide to consent* (pp. 57–67). Washington, DC: American Association on Mental Retardation.

United Nations, General Assembly (2001, December 19). *Res. 56/168 Ad hoc Committee appointed to draft proposed "International Convention on the Protection and Promotion of the Rights and Dignity of Persons with Disabilities."* New York and Geneva: Author.

Young Adult Institute. (2003). *Tool for assessing informed sexual consent through an evaluation of responsible sexual behavior.* New York: Author.

10

Managing the Risks Associated with Sexual Activity

John Rose and Melissa Rennie

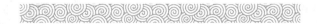

Those who provide and receive supports are migratory beings, always seeking a better balance and a more nourishing environment in which interdependence, choice, self-determination, and the right to risks can flourish.

Citizens with disabilities yearn for education, communication, participation, and the enjoyment that derives from experiencing the opportunities inherent in being members of a community. For each new activity, consumers, providers, and other stakeholders need to assess the level of desire to participate, the degree of risk involved, the ability to understand the risk, and the willingness to assume responsibility for it, and they need to arrange for appropriate supports to manage that risk. The public often demands that stakeholders also *justify the reasonableness* of their desire to pursue basic needs. Whether through indifference or deliberate attempts to exclude people with differences, society continually interposes objections grounded in misinformation between citizens with disabilities and their right to engage in the diverse activities that society itself has defined as necessary to a life of quality and fulfillment.

Through extraordinary efforts by self-advocates and other stakeholders, the public is acquiring at least an *intellectual* acceptance of the fact that citizens with disabilities have the right to live and work independently, to enjoy leisure activities, and to take advantage of educational opportunities. Members in the general public are gradually beginning to see that all individuals derive satisfaction from the same sources and that everyone is entitled access to those sources.

Only the frontiers of love, intimacy, and sexuality remain somewhat out of bounds for individuals with disabilities. This chapter will identify some of the obstacles that stand between people with disabilities and their pursuit of healthy sexual expression and the impact that these obstacles have on liability and other legal issues, including public perceptions, overprotective families, and undertrained staff. It will also examine the risks that people with intellectual and developmental disabilities and their supporters may encounter, such as unwanted pregnancies, sexually transmitted diseases (STDs), and claims of abuse, assault, and negligence. It will cover some risk management remedies that consumers and providers can employ to overcome, or at least manage, risks and obstacles. This chapter will also illustrate the premise that failing to address the issue of sexuality in all its complexities only exacerbates the risks usually associated with sexual activities, and may actually increase the risks to citizens with disabilities.

FACTORS INFLUENCING SOCIAL ACCEPTANCE

The notion that people with disabilities are sexual beings is rarely considered or discussed among members of the public, among families of many citizens with disabilities, and even among many individuals with disabilities themselves. When the topic does arise, however, it usually bursts over us in a torrent of hysteria and crisis, such as when a person with an intellectual or developmental disability has been involved in a sexual assault or other tragic incident. It is an area rife with frustrations, unreasonable prejudices, and avoidable tragedies.

Historically, there have been few realistic portrayals of people with intellectual or developmental disabilities. Misleading extremes have ranged from the helpless, child-like character to the dangerous sexual predator. In more recent times, the entertainment and news media have tried to generate more truthful coverage and more genuine characters. Knowing that people with disabilities love, have relationships, and have a right to sexual expression is a milestone in the development of our understanding of our selves and our role in supporting those with disabilities.

Ailey, Marks, Crisp, and Hahn (2003) stated that

> Persons with intellectual or developmental disabilities report having the same dreams and sexual desires as do their nondisabled peers. Nevertheless, they continue to be held to rigid standards of sexual morality and receive messages from families, professionally and society that marriage, children, and an active sexual life are forbidden. (p. 239)

They also stated

> Individuals must receive education and training . . . beginning in infancy and extending their sexuality requires the presence of several factors: developing a positive self-esteem, making choices, giving consent, receiving information, experiencing mutuality, experiencing pleasure, and having legal recourse if they are abused. (p. 239)

Perceptions

Education, culture, and experience are among the strongest influences on how provider agencies, consumers, family members, and the public perceive the issue of sexuality and disability. Together, they define the boundaries of perception.

The more limited a person's education and experience, the narrower and more distorted the person's perceptions will be. Agencies, the public, families, and consumers all have fears and concerns about sexuality and disability that are grounded in education, culture, and experience. For providers, recognizing those fears and their sources is a vital first step in accepting the challenge to manage the risks associated with sexual activity. The stronger the cultural values, the more carefully change agents must act in hoeing common ground where new ideas about relationships and sexuality can take root.

Agency Perceptions

Organizations that support people with intellectual and developmental disabilities have the tremendous challenge of balancing choice and risk, and protecting clients from harm while enhancing their right to express themselves. Although an agency's mission statement may include an "official" perspective on choice and opportunity, when it comes to sexual expression, there may well be as many views as there are staff members. Personal views, if not tempered by one's personal environment, education, training, and policy, may interfere with the personal freedom of those served. The agency is responsible for welding those many staff views into a unified approach to education, opportunity, and risk management for physical and emotional intimacy.

The fear of liability for allowing a person to experience opportunities to grow, should that experience result in harm to that individual, may also taint an agency's perception. Concerns about agency liability can affect how an organization supports someone. An agency's failure to address the issue of sexuality is also a liability and is in itself dangerous. A wiser course, in terms of consumer benefit and quality of service, is to engage in risk management practices that create policies, procedures, and opportunities that relate to sexuality and physical intimacy and incorporate the principles of individual risk preparedness and assessment.

Public Perceptions

In 1989, a group of male high school athletes from Glen Ridge, New Jersey, all with histories of sexually aggressive behavior, was accused of sexually assaulting a 17-year-old female student who was labeled as "retarded."

The incident matched the profile of acquaintance rape, but the legal professionals sidestepped that straightforward approach. The prosecution instead worked to prove that the victim was "mentally defective" and incapable of giving consent, while still preserving her credibility as a witness on her own behalf. The defense tried to discredit her testimony, yet convince a jury that she did not have mental retardation and was therefore competent to have given consent to all that was done to her, including being sexually assaulted with a broom, a baseball bat, and other objects.

The victim's character and competence were needlessly and relentlessly scrutinized. Both sides paraded expert witnesses who presented their opinions as facts about the plaintiff's mental capacity or lack of it, the nature of her disability, and, in flagrant disregard of the rape-shield laws, even her sexual history. Public attitude to the sentences of jail time meted out reflected the values that prevailed during the trial. In his post-sentencing research of the Glen Ridge case, Sobsey (1994) found that

> [E]ight times as many people thought a suspended sentence was adequate when the crime victim was described as having a developmental disability, and almost twice as many people felt that jail time should be required when the victim was described [as a professional] without a disability. In addition, when jail time was recommended, the average sentence was shorter for the crime when it was committed against a victim with a disability. (p. 7)

How could public education have led the lawyers, judge, and jury to a guilty verdict without sacrificing the victim's privacy rights and dignity? What public relations strategies might thwart the public's tendency to disregard the civil and human rights of a person with a disability in proportion to that disability, or for the benefit of a person without disabilities? What types of support or intervention could stop future cases of this type from turning on the issue of intellectual capacity and confine them to the primary issue of sexual assault? Whose voices would the public hear most clearly, those of self-advocates, or direct support professionals and experts in the field, or would it depend on the audience? How?

Family Perceptions

Sometimes, family members of individuals with disabilities present the greatest obstacles for citizens with disabilities who strive to develop a positive sense of their own sexuality. Lack of understanding or the tendency to overprotect may lead family members to unreasonable expectations or extreme reactions. In his essay titled "Self-Determination," Michael Kennedy wrote, "By not letting someone take a chance, professionals and parents make the biggest mistake they can make, because before a person becomes self-determining they've got to go through some trials and tribulations of just life itself, like anybody else" (Kennedy, 1996, p. 48).

As reported in the May 2000 TASH newsletter, some physicians may encourage parents to believe that children who require total care are automatically exempted from the risks and unable to experience the rewards of sexual activity (Hingsburger & Tough, 2000). One mother, for example, reported that her physician told her that her child's sexual organ was just a "flap of flesh." Parents of children with less significant disabilities may recognize the risks related to sexual activity, but they often steer their children away from intimate relationships out of fear and the belief that their children's abilities cannot accommodate the risks or dynamics of personal relationships. Those approaches are neither safe nor realistic. The consequences of failing to acknowledge and respond to sexuality can affect the well being of the consumer, the family, the agency, or all three.

In the same newsletter, the father of a young man with disabilities was quoted as saying, "I think I denied my son the opportunity to be with others who have disabilities and in that way, I could keep him celibate" (Hingsburger & Tough, 2000). He went on to explain that because he denied his son the opportunity to develop socialization skills, his son now acts in a sexual manner toward his mother and sister, the only women with whom he has been allowed to develop relationships.

Similarly, Leslie Walker-Hirsch reported that she had evaluated several individuals whose families expressed great concern about their child's sexually inappropriate behavior toward family members (personal communication, December, 2005). Frequently, the children had very limited social contacts with peers on account of inappropriate sexual behavior. Unfortunately, the families and schools had dealt with these inappropriate sexual expressions primarily by isolating the children from others, reducing the amount of independence for the children, and providing intense criticism of the children. The more inappropriate and frequent the sexual expressions became, the less social opportunity the children were afforded, the more independence that was lost, and the more virulent the criticism became. This cycle of social withdrawal of the children was not a successful solution to inappropriate sexual expressions, but in fact further limited the children's opportunities to learn adequate and age-appropriate coping strategies for expressing sexual feelings for another person, differentiate family members from peers who may welcome this kind of attention and education, and practice gaining control over the expression of sexual urges that are not tolerated in a particular setting.

> A recent lawsuit revolved around Ann, a young woman with an intellectual disability who was introduced to, and dated, a friend of her roommate's boyfriend. A relationship developed, which included safe, consensual sex. Ann happily told her sister that she had a boyfriend. Her sister was horrified to learn that Ann was engaging in sex and was sure that she had been coerced in some way. Because Ann has an intellectual disability, her sister could only perceive her as a victim, so "on Ann's behalf," her sister filed rape charges against the young man. Although this particular case ended without a conviction, families, juries, and lawyers (drawn from a public that is usually undereducated in this area) are often eager to *criminalize* one of the partners in such a relationship. Even though they may be well intentioned, they are rarely well informed.
>
> In their zealous but misdirected efforts to "help and protect" people with disabilities, families instead often minimize their humanity, deprive them of their rights, and further isolate them. Consider the consequences of a guilty verdict in the scenario just described. A guilty verdict based on Ann's "lack of capacity" could have made it illegal for *anyone to ever engage in sex with her again.* How would family education have helped Ann's sister to gain a more realistic view of Ann's *abilities* and be more respectful of her rights? What kind of early interventions would have helped Ann assert, to her sister, her right to choose? What risks did Ann manage successfully? Whose voice would be most effective in educating family members? How might agencies meet their responsibilities as drivers of positive change for consumers without overstepping the role of *parens patriae.*
>
> How can agencies act as buffers between consumers and their family members who may overreact to age-typical sexual interest? How might an agency encourage dialogue between parents whose children have developed intimate relationships and parents who wish to prevent their children from having access to the necessary education to experience this aspect of adult life with the least risk possible? How will the missed opportunity affect the person's quality of life?

Consumer Perceptions

Consider the victim's testimony in the Glen Ridge case mentioned previously. She testified that she thought the boys were her friends. She was concerned about them and was afraid to resist their sexual aggression because "they would think (she) didn't like them." In this handful of facts, we find significant support for the premise that people with disabilities are limited and at risk not because of their disabilities but because of societal restrictions that drive them toward emotional, educational, and experiential poverty. The risks related to isolation, loneliness, minimal inclusion, and lack of familiarity with choice might be greater than those related to physical or mental impairment, or to engaging in safe, consensual sex.

Human beings typically yearn to exchange loving, physical contact. Yet individuals who spend a significant portion of their lives in institutional or closely managed settings seldom experience the daily physical expressions of affection that abound in a family setting. States such as New York limit touching between caregivers and those with a developmental disability and between peers with intellectual disabilities. Because the ability to consent to sexual expression with another person is often undetermined, touch is limited to hand holding, friendly hugging, and chaste kissing (Howe, 1993, draft). Most of their experiences in appropriate touching is of a functional nature, such as receiving assistance in bathing and dressing. These restrictions on touching place individuals with disabilities in a consistently passive role and leaves their need for meaningful, expressive contact unfulfilled. Even in more natural settings, guidance in developing intimate relationships and healthy sexual habits is either minimal or overlooked, limiting self-awareness and self-expression. These restrictions blur the line between healthy and unhealthy relationships, or between appropriate and inappropriate touching. These shortcomings are environmental, not personal.

Behaviorist Sean Gerow said

> Relationships are complex levels of emotions at times filled with extreme happiness and at other times great sadness. People with developmental disabilities all too often experience only the sadness of the relationship. We must work together to insure that individuals fully understand what it means to be in love and to experience all that the relationship has to offer, including sexual experiences, in a manner appropriate for the individual. (personal communication, 2003)

Did the Glen Ridge victim's vulnerability really stem from a perceived intellectual disability or was it caused by an *environmental* disability that left her with a diminished sense of personal safety and choice and an overdeveloped wish to "please" others regardless of her own discomfort? How could appropriate sex education and greater exposure to *managed* risks have helped the victim recognize and avoid inappropriate advances? What types of early childhood education could encourage self-awareness and self-esteem and discourage the need to "people please"? What sorts of experiences and socialization supports during puberty could help individuals with disabilities enforce boundaries and develop decision-making skills and the appropriate means to achieve intimacy and express their sexuality? How can supporters help individuals with disabilities distinguish between affection, intimacy, and sex, and fulfill those needs and avoid exploitation? Whose voices would be most effective in speaking to consumers about different issues and at various stages of development?

Roles

Each of these perceptions generates obstacles and greatly influences the significant roles that agencies, staff, families, and consumers have to play in overcoming them. The agency is the origination point, for it must unite all stakeholders in pursuit of the common goal, using methods upon which all agree. While the family may have substantial legal rights as guardians of minors or those who do not have sufficient capacity, a direct support professional (DSP) is often responsible for day-to-day care.

Family and agency groups may need help in reconciling their roles, which sometimes seem contradictory. It is well documented that consumers with intellectual disabilities are actually taught to be compliant toward authority figures (Finlay & Lyons, 2002). The staff, although protective and nurturing to the individuals they serve, tend to place themselves more in a parental/authority role, rather than a supportive one. Consumers can and must be able to exercise their ability to assume the role of decision maker on their own behalf. When a consumer is provided with the opportunity to see and experience the various options that are available in any given situation and get information about the outcomes that are likely to be the result of making that choice, they become better able to exercise decision making and establish a preference that is based upon personal values, likes and dislikes, and individual goals. The compliant consumer and the protective staff member may need support from family members, agency administrators, clinicians, and others for replacing "learned" passive or compliant behavior with behavior driven by choice and responsibility.

The Agency's Role

In order to fulfill their mission to support consumers, staff, and family as they safely traverse this new frontier, agencies need to construct policies and procedures that chart a path through the issues of competency, consent, risk assessment, education, risk management, and staff training as they relate to sexuality. In order to do so, the agency should assemble a committee on sexuality that includes consumers, self-advocates, DSPs, parents, legal support, board members, clinicians, and management. Including such members in the committee is the best way to ensure that the agency's policies and procedures regarding the above issues are legally sufficient, address the priorities of all parties, and support the agency's mission to promote growth, choice, and safety.

Agencies should consider and implement these six important aspects of a sexual abuse prevention program:

1. Policies and procedures

2. Individual assessments to determine capacity

3. Staff, consumer, and family education

4. Monitoring

5. Evaluation

6. Establishment of an ethics or human rights committee

The lack of a formal abuse prevention program with policies that define protocols confuse staff, create an atmosphere with lack of support, and allow potential exploitation.

During a telephone interview in 2003, Perry Samowitz, a clinical sexologist and the director of Education and Training at the Young Adult Institute/National Institute for People with Disabilities (YAI/NIPD) in New York City said that at YAI/NIPD, the primary focus is on an individual's rights. Mr. Samowitz noted that the only caveat in YAI/NIPD's policy is related to safety: "if their behavior is so dangerous as to cause undue harm, abuse or exploitation to themselves or others, and they refuse to cease that behavior, their families would be notified." He also indicated that capacity weighs heavily in determining those rights. "If individuals are determined to be consenting adults, then they have the same rights as we do."

The legal question of capacity to consent to sexual contact is inextricably tied to safety, informed choice, and risk management. The definitions are vague, and they vary in degree and intention. While a simple definition might be a "knowing, intelligent, and voluntary agreement to engage in a given activity" (Kaeser, 1992), other definitions elaborate on degrees of knowing and what constitutes knowing. An individual may have knowledge of and competence in some sexual acts but not others. Another individual may understand sexual acts but may not understand the consequences. A more complete definition might state that the capacity for consent must mean *informed* consent, including access to sex education about potential risks, the ability to engage in sex responsibly, and the understanding that engaging in any sexual behavior is a matter of choice for both participants. This implies that both have adequate information about the activity, that they can express personal values and preferences, and that there is no coercion involved. Also implied is knowledge and capacity to act responsibly and respectfully toward one-self and others in relationships. Thus, a person may have the capacity to give informed consent for one type of behavior but not another. Some individuals may be able to consent to sexual activity with an individual of their choice, but may still require support in rejecting or avoiding unwanted advances.

Although each state provides legal considerations and guidelines related to consent, the programmatic specifics and the details of imple-mentation and criteria within the broader guideline limitations may be left to individual agencies. Some groups may place the highest value on personal freedom and create inclusive criteria. Others may place a high-er value on creating a risk-averse environment and implement criteria that are more heavily weighted toward protection and a less inclusive set of standards. Both the inclusive and exclusive criteria can simultaneous-ly be within the law. However, it must be stated here that simply restrict-ing a person's opportunities should not be considered an adequate risk management plan. This will be discussed more fully later in the chapter. (The subject of sexuality and the law that addresses the concerns of those with intellectual disabilities is more fully addressed in Chapter 9 of this book.)

Even *informed* sexual intimacy carries the risks of unwanted preg-nancy, discrimination based on sexual orientation, STDs, and physi-cal/mental trauma, but it also offers the possibilities of love, companionship, and physical pleasure. *Uninformed* sexual activity carries all of those risks plus a greater risk of abuse and assault, yet it offers lit-tle likelihood of the same rewards.

For providers, the risks may include lawsuits for negligence, sexual assault, rape, inappropriate behavior by staff or consumers, and the costs and time of defending suits and damage to reputation. A family faced with the cost of raising a child who is the product of a sexual encounter between their family member and a staff member or another consumer may sue the provider agency. These claims stem from some alleged fail-ure of providers to meet their responsibility to protect from harm those they support. The responsibilities that agencies undertake are typically cited in state regulations concerning licensure requirements for agen-cies that provide services to individuals with disabilities.

It is imperative that the agency's approach for each group be com-prehensive in terms of scope and balanced in terms of choice and risk management, and address the perceptions of each specific audience, that is, the public (including judges, lawyers, juries, and lawmakers), families, DSPs, and individuals with disabilities.

In each case, the "voice" must be the one that speaks with the most authority to each particular audience. For example, medical and legal experts in the field of intellectual and developmental disabilities, backed by a chorus of self-advocates, might have the loudest voice for the public while families might respond better to agency staff, self-advocates, and the consumer who is being supported. Consumers themselves may hear input from all members of their circle of support and peers who have had accrued positive histories of friendships, intimacy, and sexual activity. Elected officials may listen to voters. Although these officials are not usually agency employees, they may well be on boards of directors or advisory boards or even on ad hoc committees that agencies have created. They may even have relatives who are affected by these decisions. Elected officials do depend on the ongoing support of their constituents: The more "grass roots" the elected official, the more access that an agency is likely to have.

The agency/staff combination is the nexus in this process of education, assessment, risk management, and practical life experience. The members must draw on all available knowledge about human behavior, sex education, medical, safety, and legal issues and combine it with input from DSPs, self-advocates, families, and persons served. They must then rechannel that information at the speed and in the direction best suited to the abilities and interests of each person served.

The Direct Support Professional's Role

Vital to the quality of outcomes for the person supported is the quality of the person(s) providing the supports. In his book, *Violence and Abuse in the Lives of People with Disabilities* (1994), Richard Sobsey noted the importance of staffing in building safer service environments. Throughout each person's journey on the road toward self-determination, the DSP's role is pivotal in gathering and presenting information, helping consumers identify and express their preferences, and helping to make opportunities available at each stage of development. DSPs are the liaisons between consumers, their families, program managers, and other members of the support team because of their daily proximal contact with the individuals they serve. Because of this central role, the importance of recruiting qualified, committed DSP staff cannot be over emphasized, and their influence on outcomes must not be underestimated. Braddock (2000) states that quality of service to individuals with developmental and related disabilities is "dependent on the people hired to provide those services and supports." Before DSPs can support consumers successfully in the highly personal and controversial area of sex education, however, they themselves must be fully prepared and trained.

Significant challenges to DSPs and consumers separate the dynamics of sex education from other types of education. Older consumers may have missed the natural progression of educational stages that would have matched their physical development, while staff may have to overcome personal moral, religious, or cultural reservations that might hinder them as they help consumers prepare to experience the rewards and risks of physical intimacy. A peculiar contradiction might be seen in the premise that in order to ensure every citizen's right to safely experience emotional and physical intimacy, supporters must ask those individuals to disclose and evaluate those aspects of life that are generally considered to be most private. This difficult task requires honesty, cooperation, great sensitivity, and the ability to evaluate from a safety perspective while sometimes suspending personal preferences, cultural beliefs, and/or values regarding sex. There are a number of resources that will help both staff and consumers meet these challenges.

A good starting point is the DSPs' Code of Ethics that the National Alliance for Direct Support Professionals (NADSP) offers on their website. The underlying principles of autonomy, nonmaleficence, beneficence, justice, and fidelity can help DSPs organize their goals, expectations, and obligations into a basic belief system that they can apply to their daily activities. The NADSP training program also offers scenarios in which DSPs apply this system to dilemmas regarding choice, safety, risk, and parental influence regarding sexuality. Couvhoven (2001) discusses five foundational concepts in teaching children with intellectual disabilities about sexuality.

1. Teaching about the body and how to care for it

2. Recognizing and accessing personal privacy

3. Recognizing personal space and social boundaries, including assertiveness

4. Learning social skills to counter the consequences of loneliness and isolation

5. Recognizing and preventing sexual exploitation

As Dave Hingsburger stated in a May 2002 TASH Newsletter, having boundaries and knowing how to say no, "in a non-verbal, but assertive way are two very teachable skills, even to those with significant disabilities." (These and other crucial elements of meaningful sexuality education subject elements are addressed more fully in Chapter 2.)

As illustrated in the Glen Ridge case discussed previously, individuals with intellectual and developmental disabilities are often *conditioned* to be compliant, lack opportunities to develop social skills naturally, have poor social judgment, have difficulty focusing on consequences, and are often viewed as less credible by their exploiters.

DSPs can teach children with intellectual disabilities these essential principles and bring "up to speed" older consumers who may have missed learning these protective foundation principles and must now learn them at rates and levels that are compatible with their individual capacities. These essential principles should be followed by the more sophisticated elements of adult self-care, anatomy, physiology, social skills, social opportunities, and sexual safety and competence. Regardless of age or capacity, these steps (tailored to each individual's abilities) are essential for a safe journey towards healthy expressions and acceptance of affection, friendship, emotional and physical intimacy, in addition to the prevention of abuse, assault, and exploitation.

The Family's Role

Although statistics fluctuate from study to study, all the numbers point in the same direction. Citizens with intellectual disabilities are at a markedly greater risk of being sexually abused and assaulted (Sobsey, 1994). The first step in helping families to meet their obligations in this regard is to bring them out of denial. Parents need to replace overreactions, avoidance, or lack of acknowledgment of their children's sexual maturity and education with an "eyes wide open" appraisal of the risks and how they relate to their child's circumstances, abilities, needs, available supports, and other facts.

> Consider a young woman with a mild to moderate intellectual disability. She is capable of a consensual sexual relationship with another resident at the group home where she resides, but she is not able to rear the child that is the product of that relationship. Her parents sue the home for negligence in "allowing" their daughter to become pregnant, and seek compensation for damages to recover the costs of rearing and educating their grandchild. Some family discussions and support group involvement regarding consequences might have helped this individual exercise choice regarding alternatives to pregnancy.

In his review of Melberg-Schwier's book, *Couples with Intellectual Disabilities Talk about Living and Loving* (1994), Hingsburger says,

> The book makes it clear that people with disabilities are loving people . . . not in that 'special' way . . . but in a deeply human way. It is impossible to read this book and not begin to think about the future of children with disabilities in new ways. (Brown, 1994)

Ideally, physical intimacy is not just an isolated or clinical event; rather, it should be the natural culmination of a series of social interactions that, according to Condeluci include a relationship progression from acquaintanceship to friendship, and eventually into "covenants" (Condeluci, 1998). Only parents who acknowledge and learn about their children's sexuality and all it implies will be able to help them manage the risks, exercise choices, and follow safely that blueprint for relationships.

Parental education, understanding, and teaching are precursors in the risk management continuum. The more a parent does to reinforce the concepts of self-care, privacy, boundaries, social skills, and exploitation prevention, the better equipped the individual will be to fend off risks and make healthy choices. As secondary sexual characteristics emerge, more specific and sophisticated concepts covering reproduction, adult physiology, relationships, self-esteem, social skills, and sexual competency should follow.

Parents also have major responsibilities regarding external influences and can act in the legal and political arenas to promote awareness and early intervention regarding sexual health care and education. They are voters who have the power to lobby, petition, write letters, and participate in advocacy groups. They should also inquire about the agency's policies regarding consumers' privacy (e.g., HIPAA compliance), supervision of staff and consumers, the ratios between them, incident reporting, the qualifications of staff members, and whether there are residents who have histories of sexually aggressive behavior. Parents should be signatories to plans to ensure that they stay informed of changes to their child's program and have the chance to contribute to their child's progress and safety. Documenting parental permission is also a means of sharing the responsibility and reducing agency liability for the decision to move forward with a new activity.

The ultimate goal for parents and families is informed participation in the planning and implementation of the child's program and a strong rapport among parents, supported individuals, DSPs, and other professionals.

The Consumer's Role

Self-advocates are eloquent envoys who have already demonstrated their power as lobbyists, community activists, and educators of both peer and public. They are in fact living banners in the campaign for access to education, employment, community inclusion, and other opportunities for those with developmental disabilities. Citizens with disabilities who have the capacity, information, and desire are logical choices as peer educators and public ambassadors. As members of support teams, self-advocates will bring a first-person voice and perspective to consumers who are learning how to safely experience their sexuality and assume responsibility for the consequences.

That same voice can be a valuable catalyst in motivating the public and lawmakers to meet the costs of contraception options, disease prevention, and gynecological care that are part of a comprehensive sex education program. Lawson (1997) wrote "as important as gynecological evaluation is for the developmentally disabled population, gynecological issues are not often emphasized, and reproductive health care issues are addressed even less often." From childhood on, women with intellectual disabilities must have access to routine reproductive health care and education regarding puberty, menstrual irregularities, common ailments, menopause, and contraception options. Men with intellectual disabilities have a right to information about the mechanics of puberty, contraception, and gender-specific medical conditions.

On the local level, each consumer's willingness to play an active and informed part in his or her own sexual emancipation can find expression in opportunities to identify and participate in activities that promote a free exchange of ideas, experiences, fears, and expectations. For example, discussion groups, both single and dual gender, might be helpful in confronting fears, curing misconceptions, learning dating etiquette and how to express preferences, and even improving competency. The further consumers travel in this direction, the more proficient they will become in exercising their rights and advocating on behalf of themselves and others.

Risk Management and Its Application to Sexual Activity

Risk is the chance of personal loss or injury. *Risk management* is a structured process for controlling that risk or chance of personal loss or injury (Wikipedia, 2006). Risk management typically involves four phases: identification, assessment, treatment, and monitoring. Effective risk management in the disabilities field means forming a protective shield on two fronts. First, it should guard consumers from preventable harm, and second, it should protect the agency from legal liability arising from errors, acts, or omissions resulting from negligence and other causes of action. A successful risk management program allows for risk while minimizing risk exposure.

Agency Education, Risk Management, and Sexual Activity

An agency's general risk management arsenal starts with the implementation of carefully crafted policies that define best practices in every aspect of the agency's operation. This means that risks are identified in all areas of agency operation and standards are in place for:

- employment practices
- regulatory compliance
- outcome evaluations
- staff training

- incident reporting and investigation
- building and driver safety
- purchasing adequate insurance coverage for all the agency's exposures

In 2003, The Irwin Siegel Agency (ISA) completed a 10-year analysis of large general and professional liability claims that were experienced by human service agencies throughout the United States. Its goal was to ascertain the contributing factors that led to an incident and, in turn, the loss or claim. While full explanation of these areas is indeed a monograph for another time, five strategic areas were identified as contributors to loss potential: culture, individual plan, policies and procedures, staff, and standard of care.

When a risk management philosophy is applied to a citizen served, it is known as an Individual Risk Management Process (IRMP). Many agencies do rely on some form of IRMP before proceeding with many activities, but only some have made that definitive leap between IRMPs and quality outcomes for sexual behavior.

A comprehensive policy that complies with federal and state laws and addresses all aspects and perspectives of sexual behavior is essential to the safety and health of the agency and all of its staff and consumers. In its absence, abuse may go unreported, staff may behave inappropriately with consumers, and staff may apply their personal values to situations regarding capacity, consent, and sexual behavior, all leading to confusion and inconsistencies in freedom and treatment. A comprehensive sexual abuse prevention program should include five components: policies and procedures, individual assessments, education, monitoring, and an ethics committee.

Policy components should include:

1. Recognizing and preventing sexual assault and abuse
2. Promoting responsibility and health in sexual activity
3. Right to sexual expression and voluntary sexual activity
4. "Zero tolerance"—incident reporting and review
5. Staff—boundaries, training, screening

Individual assessment should include:

1. Individual demonstrates self-protection knowledge and skills.
2. Individual demonstrates precedence in establishing and maintaining relationships with others.

3. Individual demonstrates sufficient knowledge to protect him- or herself against unwanted pregnancy.

4. Individual demonstrates sufficient knowledge to protect him- or herself against sexually transmitted diseases.

The trainer/educator should possess certain education skills that are likely to encourage individuals with disabilities to understand and retain information. They include:

- Extensive knowledge based on sexual education
- Formation and maintenance of relationships
- Ability to clarify information
- Knowledge of STIs
- Consequences of sexual expression
- Conception knowledge

The education program needs to address all areas of sexuality. Lessons should include:

- Social skills—public and private information, dating, relationships, social distance, posture
- Reproduction—anatomy, biological function, menstruation, birth control
- Prevention of sexual abuse—saying NO
- Reporting inappropriate incidents
- STDs—transmission, safer sex, abstinence
- Personal safety skills
- Self defense training
- Sexual orientation—choice regarding preference

Monitoring is a critical component of the plan, and should include the following elements:

- Develop and implement an incident management program
- Prevention—primary focus
- Screening of volunteers and employees
- Identification
- Training of all stakeholders
- Protection
- Investigation

- Report
- Respond—follow up and implement change
- Supervisory training and accountability
- Detect Abuse—protocol for response by direct care staff
- Stress management
- Mentoring staff

An ethics committee should be developed and comprised of community membership as well as staff and consumers. During this meeting, the following should occur:

- Review training and policies and procedures
- Evaluate assessment concerns
- Report to board

The Basis for Lawsuits

People can sue for many reasons related to sexual behavior, and providers need to realize this and plan accordingly. For example, consumers may impose their will on each other or be denied their right to sexual expression. Regulatory noncompliance may also lead to fines or other sanctions against the agency. The same risk management strategies that help to guard consumers and guide staff can also help to minimize the possibility of an agency being sued and help to prepare a strong defense in case of a claim.

The criteria for a successful lawsuit seem clear in theory. In order for a plaintiff to prevail, the defendant must be proven liable. To be proven liable, the following four conditions must be met:

- A **Duty** or obligation, recognized by the law, requiring the person to conform to a certain standard of conduct, for the protection of others from unreasonable risks.

- A **Failure** or **Breach** on the person's part to meet the duty; a failure to conform to a recognized standard of care.

- A reasonably close or **Causal Connection** between the conduct (breach) and the resulting injury; what is known as proximate or legal cause.

- Actual loss or **Damages** resulting from negligence. (Keeton, 1984)

In reality, the four conditions of liability can get very fuzzy when uninformed lawyers and jurors attempt to apply them to variables like intellectual capacity and informed consent. Consumers, and therefore providers, are safest when they apply the same risk management criteria consistently on both fronts. That means identifying as many risks as possible and evaluating them for severity and probability of occurrence. This may involve developing a risk management plan that includes an individual plan of protection, which may require input from a professional such as a psychologist and perhaps family members as well, and applying appropriate risk management remedies. These remedies should include education, supervision, regular evaluations and monitoring, and appropriate insurance coverage including coverage for sexual abuse and molestation.

Strictly enforcing policies related to routine documentation and meticulous reporting and investigation of incidents is crucial to defending a lawsuit. If an agency is sued or a consumer's rights are challenged, logs and other records are vital to a successful defense. Of these, records relating to the consumer's Individual Program Plan are paramount. Attorney Chris Lyons said, "Where a proper assessment (with the consumer) has been made regarding capacity and desire, and a proper plan devised regarding sexuality (training and behavior) and the plan has been properly effectuated, it can be argued that the Agency has met its duty, regardless of the actual outcome" (personal communication, 2003).

Public Education, Risk Management, and Sexual Activity

In addition to generating support for right-to-risk and self-determination, a public awareness and relations campaign is a powerful, long-term risk management tool. The public includes those who make, vote on, interpret, and enforce laws in your community. They are the teachers, doctors, jurors, and lawyers, who may, at any time, have some decision-making powers regarding an agency and those the agency serves.

Recall Ann who was discussed previously. Picture a scenario similar to Ann's in which a resident-consumer enters a relationship with a fellow resident and a family member or guardian sues the provider for negligence or sexual assault. Remember the four elements of liability: duty, breach of duty, proximate cause, and damages. As "strangers in a strange land" (the world of intellectual disabilities), uninformed lawyers, judges, and "expert" witnesses may very well decide that the facts of the case meet the legal standards for liability, find for the plaintiff, and award a large financial settlement. In addition to financial loss, the agency may lose time and productivity and suffer a tarnished reputation. A verdict in favor of the plaintiff might also negate the consumers' right to continue their intimate relationship and place a perpetual legal obligation on the agency to uphold that negation. An agency that wages a vigorous, local public education campaign is more likely to encounter lawyers, judges, and juries who recognize the right of the two consumers to enter into a consensual relationship. The risk management technique of public education may help a judge and jury to decide in favor of the agency and therefore the consumers.

Public education may also improve quality of life and safety for your consumers as they increase their participation in community life. Citizens with intellectual disabilities are entitled to experience inclusion and participation in their communities. Consumers will be purchasing goods and services from their local bus drivers, pharmacies, restaurants, hotels, and shopkeepers. They may be volunteers or employees in the community. Just as providers prepare those they support for the responsibilities of community life, they should also help the community prepare to welcome citizens with disabilities as valuable members of the community.

There is no doubt that the public believes there are differences between those who have disabilities and those who do not. Only education and inclusion will help the public understand that any differences are singular and minimal while the similarities are universal and plentiful.

Public education includes developing relationships with local media, civic organizations, schools, and religious groups who can publicize and pass along your messages of right-to-risk, inclusion, and ability to contribute. The value of a public relations staff and a program that includes self-advocates as ambassadors is immense. Agency staff, volunteers, and consumers should all be well prepared to assume the responsibilities of being envoys to the community.

Consumer Education, Risk Management, and Sexual Activity

In the context of physical intimacy, one of the *risks* might be acquiring a sexually transmitted disease. The *hazard* would be not practicing safe sex. The *severity* of the potential harm could range from a simple infection that is easily cured, to a serious, life-threatening disease. The *probability* of getting an infection is greater if one or both partners have had multiple partners with whom they did not practice safe sex.

This process of identifying the risk and related hazards, measuring its severity, and determining the probability of occurrence are the fundamentals of risk management regardless of circumstances. Parents of children without disabilities apply this risk management process routinely and often without recognizing it as such. For example, a parent might say, "At this age, my child will ride a tricycle, at this age he or she will ride a two-wheeler with training wheels, and at this age I will take the training wheels off. I will expect his or her peers to follow a similar schedule."

In the context of intellectual disabilities, the typical schedule of *physical* maturity (i.e., the emergence of secondary sexual characteristics and desires) may apply to many individuals of the same chronological age group, while the schedules for physical coordination and cognitive and emotional development may be widely divergent. This means that in addition to applying the foundations of risk management, supporters must also assess each individual's level of ability to participate in a given activity, desire to do so, understanding of the risks inherent in the activity, and willingness to assume responsibility for the risk and its consequences. Based on this assessment of choice/desire, education, and responsibility, an informed decision needs to be made to proceed, proceed with a modified version or with additional supports, to avoid the activity, or to postpone it, possibly until the individual acquires greater intermediate experience and competence. The trigger for each assessment must be the desires of the person served, and the results should always lead toward *informed* choice, *accepted* responsibility, and *managed* risk. The key to this process is the individual's care plan or support plan. It not only lays the foundation for the DSP and others, but it is also the one tool that can minimize the consumer's and the agency's exposure to risk.

It is becoming a standard risk management practice to apply these assessment criteria to personal care, coping skills, body awareness, social skills, and personal safety in this manner. The results are used to make and implement informed decisions regarding living, working, and traveling in the community. Because sexuality and intimacy involve elements from all of these areas, the following shows how preliminary assessment criteria might be formulated by pulling the relevant items from each of those areas and adapting them to reflect Couvhoven's (2001) five foundational concepts or a similar model.

These foundational concepts are the bare bones of consumer education and assessment relating to personal relationships and physical intimacy and they are vital to a successful IRMP in that context. They form the *foundation* on which each individual's program plan will be built, and it is part of the agency's mission to build upon that foundation. It is important to point out that consumer education is as vital to self-determination and safety as it is to protection and assertion of rights. In case of a claim, your consumers will be more compelling witnesses on their own behalf if they have had the benefits of honest discussions, appropriate supports, and positive life experiences. Factors in the individual risk preparedness assessment include

- Understands risks associated with activity
- Takes responsibility for risks related to the activity

- Assessment of possibility of harm occurring
- Considers severity of potential harm
- Indicates desire to participate in activity

Building a Circle of Support

There are many kinds of loving relationships, and they all vary in degree and intensity. Although most relationships may include some physical demonstrations of affection, it is worth noting that very few of them include sex as a means of expressing that love. Parental devotion, sibling love, close friendships, even pets, present opportunities to give and receive expressions of love without any sexual activity. Among those close friendships, one special one may evolve to include physical intimacy. Like opportunities to live, work, volunteer, and be fully vested members of a community, the chance for individuals with intellectual disabilities to develop naturally a spectrum of warm relationships depends on opportunities to participate and gain experience. A Circle of Support is the portal to those opportunities and experiences (Falvey et al., 1993).

A successful Circle of Support relies on total commitment to the elements of education, training, dialogue, assessment, and risk management discussed previously. Consumers, parents, and staff have well-defined roles and the tools to perform them. Consumers participate in discussions and educational groups to help them understand self-care, safety, respect, and preferences in the context of their own and others' sexuality. Parents have the benefit of mutual sharing and other forums for improving their awareness, acceptance, and communication skills regarding their children as sexual beings. Staff follow clearly articulated policies that ensure safety, quality, compliance, and consistency concerning physical intimacy among those they serve. A multi-faceted community relations and public education campaign is underway and includes a strong self-advocate presence. These components will come together to help consumers expand their awareness of self and others as emotional, physical, social, loving, and sexual beings and extend their opportunities to give and receive expressions of those feelings. As Sobsey (1994) observed, "isolation increases risk. What we are really talking about here is how to replace isolation with participation."

Six Circles

Like ripples in a pond, the Circle of Support has many rings. The stronger that first ripple is, the stronger the other rings will be and the further they will travel. The larger the circle, the smaller the risk will be to the individual. In the innermost circle are the individuals served and those few with the greatest influence and responsibility in their lives. In the words of Dr. Condeluci, they have *covenants* with the individual and might include parents and siblings. A second circle might contain *intimate friends* and a DSP or other agency staff member who has a close daily relationship with the individual. A third circle might be composed of *closest friends* and other support staff. Coworkers with whom the individual has *friendships* might occupy the fourth circle. And in the fifth circle might be *initial friends* and perhaps a health care professional with whom the individual has frequent contact or a long-term relationship. In the sixth circle are community *acquaintances.* If the inner circles are effective, they will pull some of the acquaintances inward (Condeluci, 1998).

Supporters of individuals with intellectual disabilities, particularly from the first three circles, often make up the interdisciplinary team that will help the citizen served to shape his or her support plan. Using the resources of policies, training, education, risk management, and information, the team will help the individual identify his or her desire to participate in certain activities, assess the ability to do so, and evaluate the risks associated with those activities. Guided by the results, the team will arrange for needed supports so that the individual can fulfill those desires safely and successfully. It is not enough, however, for the inner circles to master the immediate mechanics of inclusion, because the further an individual travels from the center of support, the greater the challenges, risks, and obstacles become. They must also build the bridges by which individuals cross over safely into the community.

Condeluci identifies four steps to "bridge building" into the community: Point of Connection, Venue, Elements of Culture, and Gatekeeper (Condeluci, 2002). Acquaintances may use those same bridges to join the inner circle, assume vital supporting roles in the individual's journey toward inclusion, and strengthen his or her risk management arsenal.

Obstacles to Inclusion

Logistical obstacles such as transportation, personal finances, and finding venues require practical solutions that are easy to identify but difficult to obtain. Others, like discrimination, are insidious and pervasive. Passive discrimination is about invisibility and it is all around us. It is the absence of wheelchair access at a community barbecue, a failure to invite an individual with an intellectual disability to participate in a neighborhood project, an absence of accommodation for individuals with hearing impairments at a town meeting, and ignoring someone who may be lost or in difficulty and in a consistent pattern of "forgetting to remember." Often there is nothing specifically illegal in acts of passive discrimination, and, therefore, there is no legal remedy that can be applied. Only education and experience can uproot the weeds of passive discrimination.

Active discrimination includes refusing to hire; failing to give the usual standard of service at the local department store, library, or hospital; refusing to rent an apartment; or enacting a policy based on disability rather than civil rights. Many of these examples of active discrimination do have avenues of legal redress, and sometimes it is necessary to travel them, but the process can be lengthy, inconvenient, and costly. The individual, as such, may be swept away on a tide of legalese.

As an alternative, the powerful machinery of a diversified Circle of Support is an immediate and efficient champion for the individual, which offers him or her the advantages of personal participation and opportunities for self-advocacy in overcoming those obstacles to inclusion and participation.

This is where the strength of the inner circle must begin to radiate outwards and draw members of the outer circle inward. No matter how well prepared an individual is, no matter how committed the interdisciplinary team is, and no matter how competent the DSP is, acquaintances from the outer circle must take an active interest in the individual if the individual is to achieve his or her goals of inclusion and community membership. Members of the outer circles are the "bridge" by which the individual crosses from the inner circles of family and other close supporters to the outer circle of community life.

In a way, the Circle of Support can be used as a mini-community to advance the inclusion and full community participation of an individual. Only when we consider the communities of support can we begin to frame a structure based on community theory. Condeluci (2002) articulated the following elements of community and how they can be used to develop circles:

- All communities are built from a notion of commonality. That is, the community must have an issue with which everyone agrees and around which it will rally. In the Circle of Support, this rally point would be a genuine interest in the person's inclusion.

- The next key ingredient of community is regularity, meaning that the members must come together often and keep the rally point going. Interestingly enough, when people come together frequently for one purpose, they often learn that they are linked in other ways as well. This further bonds the community members.

- As the community continues to meet, they begin to develop rituals, which are defined by behaviors that all the members begin to perform. Rituals help community members feel more comfortable and at home.

- After the community is organized, it develops a potent ingredient in the form of shared memory. This refers to the work and achievements of the community and creates a strong sense of commitment to the common goal.

- The last (but not least) important feature for the community is the members' understanding of their roles as gatekeepers. In a community, a gatekeeper is a member who offers links to other people and communities. These gatekeepers are essential to the process because they are the bankers of "social capital," which is the currency of life.

Sociologists tell us that we find "social capital" in the communities to which we belong, and this social capital helps to keep us safe and healthy because our friends watch out for us. It is a form of risk management when community members check why someone has not answered the phone, offer help if there has been a power outage, give rides to the doctor's office, and help each other avoid dangerous activities. Investments of social capital often pay dividends in reciprocity on which communities thrive.

Perhaps some individuals at an agency would like to take a ceramics class but require a little extra supervision. Others would like to join the local dance club, but the dues are more than they can manage. A few consumers want to volunteer at a nursing home, but need transportation. A couple wishes to live in their own apartment together, but it seems that no one wants to rent to them. The interdisciplinary team must convince an authority within each of these venues to lend the supported individuals some of their power to be a gatekeeper.

Maybe the ceramics teacher can ask some advanced students to buddy-up with each of the new members of the class. Perhaps the dance club will vote to accept partial dues and give the supported individuals the opportunity to work off the balance by serving refreshments or helping with mailings. Would a local taxi company pick up and drop off the volunteers at the nursing home once a week? Maybe a local realtor would be able to help the couple find an apartment.

"Small World" Research

There are probably several ways to overcome obstacles to inclusion, and finding them is a lot like playing the game "Six Degrees of Separation." Harvard social psychologist Stanley Milgram began what came to be known as "Small World Research" based on the premise that a chain of six people or less connects each of us to everyone else (Milgram, 1967). The theory spawned a hit play by John Guare, a movie, and a popular game. For those interested in creating natural opportunities to socialize, develop personal relationships, and extend a Circle of Support, it is a valuable tool for both reciprocity and risk management that is well worth exploring.

The ceramics teacher, for example, may be the DSP's neighbor. It turns out that the secretary of the dance club has a daughter who goes to school with the sibling of one of the consumers. The taxi driver has a relative in the nursing home. He would like to know someone is visiting her once a week. The couple's job coach is a member of a local civic organization. One of the other members is a realtor who wants to run for local office and would welcome a chance to "get involved" by fighting what appears to be a case of discrimination. The two of them also convince the organization to help the couple get set up in their new apartment. Regardless of their motives, each of these individuals became a gatekeeper. They invested social capital in consumers, some of whom were able to reciprocate with their own investments.

From a risk management perspective, what are the possible outcomes without gatekeepers? Without their mentors, the individuals in the ceramics class are at greater risk from the sharp tools and high kiln temperatures. They will learn less, and without that bridge to the rest of the class, they may tend to stick together and not interact with this group of strangers. The dancers find the only alternative to the dance club is a local bar that has live music. While they are there, a fight breaks out and one of them is injured. If the visitors cannot get to the nursing home, the community will lose the benefit of their contribution, and the residents of the nursing home will be deprived of the only visitors many of them might have. The couple is denied their dream of making a home together, and because they must continue to pay two rents, they cannot afford to enroll in a continuing education class that would enhance their employment opportunities.

SUMMARY

The self-advocacy movement has inspired individuals to challenge more in their lives and to replace the traditional service delivery system with a consumer directed service delivery system. *This trend may shift the nature but not the weight of the providers' responsibilities.* Families and/or consumers may assume more responsibilities and control in choosing paths and supports, but the agency remains the focal point from which those paths emanate, and the agency retains the responsibility for all that implies. To attain the ultimate goal of inclusion, consumers need to be S.A.F.E.R. This requires an interdependence of:

System

Advocacy

Family and Friends

Environment

Risk Management

That citizens with disabilities have not learned the life skills necessary for community inclusion and DSPs have not learned how to teach them is a function of omission, not of disability, particularly for older citizens who grew up in a system driven by a philosophy of "manage and control." Failure to respond to those shifts with more sophisticated approaches to risk management, staff training, and consumer education will leave consumers open to greater probability of harm and agencies open to greater likelihood of claims for negligence. Failure to facilitate opportunities for consumers to put that knowledge to practical use is to deny them their fundamental human rights.

This education and assistance does not differ significantly from that which most families supply as a matter of course. No one is born knowing how to make friends, ride a bike, or balance a checkbook. Learning how to develop loving relationships that lead to physical intimacy is just one more rite of passage that most parents and educational systems help children traverse in the natural course of growing up. What toddler knows instinctively the difference between appropriate and inappropriate touching? Does any child know, without being told, not to impose his or her will on others? What adolescent is able to define and enforce dating boundaries without guidance? Can any adult cultivate meaningful relationships or enjoy the rewards and responsibilities of adulthood without opportunities to participate in community life? Parents' duty to teach respect and responsibility toward self and others does not change when their son or daughter has an intellectual disability, nor does their obligation to maintain the "natural" environment that a child without disabilities would enjoy as a matter of course.

Given the opportunities to learn through education and experience, citizens with disabilities can enjoy lives of contribution and participation driven by choice and grounded in self-determination. With commitment, understanding, and training, providers can help them achieve those ideals.

REFERENCES

Ailey, S.H., Marks, B.A., Crisp, C., & Hahn, J.E. (2003). Promoting sexuality across the life span for individuals with intellectual and developmental disabilities. *Nursing Clinics of North America, 33*(2), 229–252.

Braddock, D. (2000). *Developmental disabilities in North Dakota: The year 2000.* Report commissioned by The Arc, Upper Valley, North Dakota.

Brown, G. (1994). *Human sexuality handbook: Guiding people toward positive expressions of sexuality.* Springfield, MA: Association for Community Living.

Condeluci, A. (2002). *Cultural shifting: Community leadership and change.* St. Augustine, FL: Training Resource Network, Inc.

Condeluci, A. (1998). *Interdependence: The road to community* (2nd ed.). Boca Raton, FL: CRC Press.

Couvenhoven, T. (2001). Unpublished lecture from the 2001 Down Syndrome Family Conference, Syracuse, NY.

Falvey, M., Forest, M., Pearpoint, J., & Rosenberg, R. (1993). *All my life's a circle: Using the tools.* Toronto: Inclusion Press.

Finlay, W.M., & Lyons, E. (2002, February). Acquiescence in interviews with people who have mental retardation. *Mental Retardation, 40*(1), 14–29.

Hill Kennedy, C., & Niederbuhl, J. (2001). Establishing criteria for sexual consent capacity. *American Journal on Mental Retardation, 106*(6), 503–510.

Hingsburger, D. (1990). *The human sexuality handbook.* Springfield, MA: The Association for Community Living.

Hingsburger, D., & Tough, S. (2000, May). Health sexuality: Attitudes, systems, and policies in research and practice for persons with severe disabilities. *TASH Newsletter, 27*(1).

Howe, E. (1993). *Guidelines on sexual contact* (draft). New York: State Office of Mental Retardation and Developmental Disabilities.

Kaeser, F. (1992). Can people with severe mental retardation consent to mutual sex? *Sexuality and Disability, 10,* 33–42.

Keeton, W.P. (Ed.). (1984). *Prosser and Keeton's hornbook on torts.* (5th ed.). St. Paul, MN: West Publishing Co.

Kennedy, M. (1996). Self-Determination and trust: My experiences and thoughts. In D.J. Sands and M.L. Wehmeyer, *Self-Determination across the life span: Independence and choice for people with disabilities.* Baltimore: Paul H. Brookes Publishing Co.

Lawson, I.D., and Elkins, T.E. (1997). Gynecologic concerns. In S.M. Pueschel & M. Sustrova (Eds.), *Adolescents with Down syndrome.* Baltimore: Paul H. Brookes Publishing Co.

Melberg-Schwier, K.M. (1994). *Couples with intellectual disabilities talk about living and loving.* Rockville, MD: Woodbine House.

Milgram, S. (1967). The small world problem. *Psychology Today, 2,* 60–67.

Sobsey, R. (1994). *Violence and abuse in the lives of people with disabilities.* Baltimore: Paul H. Brookes Publishing Co.

Wikipedia. (n.d.). Risk management. Retrieved March 3, 2006, from www.en.wikipedia.org/wiki/Risk_management

ORGANIZATIONS, RESOURCES, AND RECOMMENDED PUBLICATIONS

National Dissemination Center for Children with Disabilities

Post Office Box 1492, Washington, DC 20013

1-800-695-0285 (Voice/TTY)

e-mail: nichcy@aed.org

URL: http://www.nichcy.org/

National Alliance of Direct Support Professionals
Post Office Box 13315, Minneapolis, MN 55414
URL: http://www.NADSP.org

New York State Commission on Quality of Care for Persons with Disabilities
401 State Street, Schenectady, NY, 12305
1-800-624-4143
URL: http://www.webmaster@cqcapd.state.ny.us

The Arc of the United States
1010 Wayne Avenue, Suite 650, Silver Spring, MD 20910
301-565-3842
email: info@thearc.org
URL: http://www.thearc.org

Center on Human Policy
Syracuse University
805 South Crouse Avenue, Syracuse, NY 13244
1-800-894-0824, TTY 315-443-4355
URL: http://thechp.syr.edu

The Center for Research for Women with Disabilities
1709 Dryden Road, Suite 725, Houston, TX 77030
1-800-44-CROWD
URL: http://www.bcm.edu/crowd/

Frontline Initiative
Post Office Box 13315, Minneapolis, MN 55414
612-624-0060
email: ander447@tc.umn.edu

iCan, Inc.
870 Bowers Street, Birmingham, MI 48009
1-877-ASK-iCan
email: services@icanonline.net

TASH (formerly The Association for Persons with Severe Handicaps) Newsletter
29 W. Susquehanna Ave. Suite 210, Baltimore, MD 21204
410-828-8274
email: info@tash.org

IV

Treatment Issues

11

OB-GYN Care for Females with Intellectual Disabilities

Mary E. White and Stuart A. Lustberg

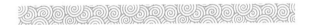

Women with intellectual disabilities have the same reproductive health issues as women without intellectual disabilities. Menstrual problems, sexuality and intimacy concerns, pregnancy and childbearing, gender-specific health risks (e.g., cancers of the breast and pelvis), and issues of aging bodies affect all women. However, women with intellectual disabilities have specific concerns and diverse needs, which warrant caring attention.

Women with intellectual disabilities may never receive quality health care for a variety of reasons. These may include:

- lack of access to services with personnel skillful in the provision of care to women with intellectual disabilities
- structural barriers for women who have concomitant physical needs (e.g., wheelchair access, adjustable gynecologic tables, mammogram machines that can accommodate to physical differences)
- care not coordinated between multiple health care specialists
- financial limitations, especially with the new managed care approach to medical reimbursement
- health care provider insensitivities or negative attitudes
- health care providers who focus on the disability rather than preventive health care needs
- limitations in the ability of a woman or her caregiver to understand and communicate her health needs (Association of State and Territorial Health Officials [ASTHO], 2003; Welner, 1999)

Health care should be a right afforded to all. In 2000, the U.S. Department of Health and Human Services (DHHS) issued *Healthy People 2010* (DHHS, 2000), a comprehensive federal agenda outlining directives and health goals for the American populace. For the first time, this report addressed the needs of people with disabilities in a separate section. The declared aims in the report are "to promote health, well-being, independence, productivity and full societal participation of people with disabilities and to lower their incidence and severity of secondary conditions." "Secondary conditions" mean health problems that arise in relation to the disability. For example, lack of skills in negotiating healthy interpersonal relationships and being dependent on others for personal care are factors that make a person with an intellectual disability more vulnerable to sexual abuse, thus, sexually transmitted diseases (STDs) can become a secondary condition.

Research shows that individuals with disabilities use the health care system less frequently than individuals in the general population, and women with disabilities are less likely to have routine preventive screening (e.g., Pap tests, mammograms; ASTHO, 2003; Tezzoni, McCarthy, Davis, Harris, & O'Day, 2001). Preventive care, however, is a hallmark of quality health care. Screening for indicators of potential problems and early disease with appropriate intervention, vaccination schedules, health education, and guidance all help to ensure a higher quality of life. People with disabilities present an array of challenges necessitating a responsive health care system to meet their needs.

Current guidelines issued by the American College of Obstetricians and Gynecologists (ACOG) advise that females 21 years of age or older should see a gynecologist, or sooner if they are sexually active. Someone who is having pelvic discomfort or difficulties with her periods, however, should visit a gynecologist sooner (ACOG, August 2003). Again, it is important to individualize these recommendations. Similarly, earlier initiation of gynecologic care is justified if an individual finds herself in situations that may be associated with sexual vulnerability or facing opportunities for consensual sexual relationships to develop. Sexually active adolescents and women need gynecologic visits annually with pap smears taken every 1–3 years.

Women ages 40 and older should be referred for screening mammograms yearly. Mammography screening is advised earlier in women with abnormal clinical breast exams or strong family histories of breast cancer; however, screening is not usually recommended prior to age 35 because mammograms have been found to be less accurate prior to this age (ACOG, April 2003).

Family members and other caregivers usually have the greatest responsibility to seek quality health care for women with intellectual disabilities. This responsibility may be overwhelming and stressful, especially in the context of prior negative encounters. The aim of this chapter is to present strategies that can smooth the way for the provision of higher-quality, multidisciplinary health care that is better accepted by a patient and her family.

It may be challenging to locate a health care provider with the sensitivity and willingness to provide careful and caring gynecological services. Probably the best route is "word of mouth" referral. The local chapter of The Arc, formerly called The Association of Retarded Citizens or The UCP, formerly called United Cerebral Palsy mental health associations, and community organizations that attend to needs of people with developmental or intellectual disabilities can be good referral sources. Planned Parenthood affiliates can be another excellent resource. Family members and other caregivers may find it helpful to use their computers to learn more about or to query various organizations.

The key to ensuring good care is to be able to provide the OB-GYN health care practitioner (e.g., physician, nurse, nurse practitioner) with as much information as possible regarding a patient's health history. Ideally, the woman should be knowledgeable about her body and her disability and should be the one giving the information to the provider. A woman's ability to do this, however, will vary greatly depending on her language development, maturity, emotional stability, and understanding. While obtaining information regarding a woman's medical history and symptoms can be difficult for caregivers of a resident who has limited family contact and is unable to speak for herself, it can not be stressed enough how important a role the history plays in determining the best plan of care. A good history, more than anything else, often leads to the diagnosis or reassurance that everything is fine. If a woman has significant disabilities, caregivers have a special responsibility for providing as much information as is possible and need to accompany the woman to her visit.

It is important to collect and keep accurate information regarding an individual's medical history. It is especially important if the person has an intellectual or developmental disability because her ability to remember and communicate significant and relevant medical information may be limited, and she may have had many different caregivers over the course of her life. She may not know which life events, medications, or previous medical procedures have significance in a specific health care situation. In order to assure the best treatment, accurate documentation provides a good first step! The following sections serve as a guide to collecting this pertinent medical history.

PERSONAL AND FAMILY HISTORY

It is helpful to health care providers if patients and/or caregivers can obtain and bring prior records, even of routine health care, to the visit. Examples of helpful past medical information include:

1. What led to the patient's intellectual disability?
2. Does she have any chronic medical illnesses, such as hypertension, asthma, epilepsy, or heart problems?
3. Has she been hospitalized? Why? When?
4. Has she had any surgeries? What type? When?
5. Has she had any complications related to past surgeries? What type? When?
6. Has she received blood transfusions? When?
7. Has she been diagnosed with any psychiatric illnesses? What type? When?
8. Is she up-to-date on routine vaccinations?
9. Is there any record of a positive tuberculin skin test?

Usually, a family history pertains to the woman's parents, siblings, grandparents, and children (if any). Obtaining a family history enables the provider to tailor appropriate screening tests for the individual woman. For example, if a woman has breast cancer in her family, determining the best screening methods and intervals depends on how she is related to the person with breast cancer, how many relatives have or had breast cancer, the age of onset of the cancer, and if there were other cancers in the family, specifically, ovarian or colon. Knowing the occurrence of other familial incidences of mental retardation or illness or birth defects also is useful to health care providers in helping to determine the likelihood of risk to a woman's offspring.

Menstruation

Keeping a menstrual calendar (noting the dates and lengths of bleeding episodes) and bringing it to the medical visit provides the health care provider with useful information. Depending on a woman's ability, it may be necessary for caregivers to check the patient's laundry (e.g., towels, underwear) to determine when or if she is bleeding. The caregiver should be able to assist in answering the following questions about the woman's menses to determine the normalcy of the patient's reproductive health.

1. At what age did the patient get her first period?
2. When was her last menstruation?
3. How many days does she bleed? How heavy or light? (It can help to estimate how many pads or tampons are soaked in a day, if the individual is able to tell the physician, or the caregiver is able to get this information.)
4. Does she have bad cramps or pass big clots?
5. Does she take any medications (even over-the-counter) for her periods?
6. Has there been a recent change in her menstrual pattern?
7. Does she have cyclic symptoms such as headaches or mood swings?
8. Does she experience bleeding or spotting between periods?
9. For older women, has she had bleeding or spotting since menopause? (This can be a sign of cancer.)

Sexual Activity

Sexual activity is an area that family members, caregivers, and even health care providers often do not feel comfortable addressing, yet it has many ramifications for the quality of life of the woman with an intellectual disability. A skillful provider will interview a woman in private about her sexual life and will tailor his or her language chosen to the level of the woman's understanding. Questions pertaining to a woman's sexual activity may include the following:

1. What does the patient know about sex?
2. Is she currently or has she been sexually active with a partner? Were these experiences pleasurable for her?
3. Has sex been forced upon her?
4. Does she understand what she is doing?
5. Does she use any protection against pregnancy or STDs?
6. Does she need birth control or instruction on its use?
7. Does she have/need access to condoms or instructions on condom use?
8. Has she used contraception? If so, which methods, and did she have difficulties with their use or side effects?

9. Does she have a history of any sexually transmitted infections?

10. Are there symptoms she has that could indicate an STD, such as unusual vaginal discharge; itching, odors, sores, bumps, or rashes in the genital area; painful urination, or lower abdominal or pelvic pain?

Health care providers have ethical and legal responsibilities to notify the appropriate authorities (i.e., child or adult protective services) if they have reason to suspect that a patient is the victim of physical, emotional, or sexual abuse or neglect. The presence of an STD is usually reportable to the local health department.

Pregnancy

If a woman with an intellectual disability has been pregnant, information regarding the course and outcome of the pregnancy, or pregnancies, is important, especially if current or future childbearing is likely. Questions pertaining to a woman's pregnancy history may include the following:

1. Has the patient had healthy pregnancies? Did she have any miscarriages or abortions? What happened?

2. What kind of delivery was performed (normal vaginal, forceps, Cesarean)?

3. Did she have any prenatal complications, such as high blood pressure, preeclampsia, diabetes, bleeding, or hospitalizations?

4. Was the baby healthy at birth? Is the child still alive?

5. How did it go after the baby was born?

6. Has she parented the child? If not, where is the child now?

7. How has she been as a parent (i.e., did she get postpartum depression, did child protective services get involved, is the baby in good health)?

8. What kind of social support does she have?

The fear of social stigma often leads women with intellectual disabilities and their families to withhold information about prior pregnancies, especially ones that ended in abortion or adoption. Withholding such information, however, limits the ability of the OB-GYN health care provider to foresee potential future problems.

Margaret is 29 years old and has a mild intellectual disability. She is pregnant and has been referred to Dr. L. for prenatal care. Margaret has a boyfriend who she met in the residential facility where they both live. She goes to the sheltered workshop with him on the bus daily, and, unbeknownst to the staff, they have become sexually intimate. Margaret and her boyfriend did not use any birth control, and now she is 18 weeks pregnant. Her mother placed her in this facility 2 years ago when her own health became frail. Margaret and her mother are opposed to abortion. The staff member that brought Margaret to see Dr. L. was unaware that Margaret had given birth to a stillborn baby at 7 months of pregnancy when Margaret was 16 years old and that she had two miscarriages in subsequent years. If Dr. L. had this information, he could begin careful monitoring of Margaret's cervix to check for signs of impending miscarriage or preterm delivery. If the doctor did not have that information, this could lead to a failure to detect a condition that could be treatable.

Medications

Patients, family members, and health care providers need to know the names and dosages of medications patients are taking in order to avoid harmful interactions with other medications or procedures that may be prescribed. Most providers encourage patients to bring current medication logs or even the prescription bottles. Oftentimes, certain medications (e.g., anticonvulsants, psychotropic medications) can be the cause of menstrual irregularities (e.g., heavy vaginal bleeding), urinary problems, or other medical problems (e.g., early bone loss [osteoporosis], anemia). Any over-the-counter drugs or herbal or vitamin supplements should be listed as well. Lastly, it is important for health care providers to ask about any known allergies to medications, foods, or other substances, as further exposure to such substances can be life threatening.

Gina is 35 years old and has been referred to a gynecologist, Dr. K., by her primary care provider who is contemplating a urology consult as well. Since a traumatic brain injury, Gina has depression along with memory lapses and difficulty with motor coordination. While waiting in the exam room for her evaluation, Gina gets dressed and subsequently undressed several times in order to use the bathroom repeatedly. When Dr. K. enters the exam room, Gina smells of urine, and the examining table paper is wet and torn. When reviewing her medication list, Dr. K. notes that one of the antidepressants Gina takes can cause urinary frequency and incontinence. Dr. K. contacted her psychiatrist to discuss switching to a different antidepressant. Once Gina began taking a new medication, she no longer suffered from urinary problems and did not need to see a urologist.

ESTABLISHING COMPETENCY AND GUARDIANSHIP

In order for individuals with intellectual disabilities to access any medical services, the issues of competency and guardianship must first be established. Is the patient able to consent for her own care? This means determining if she has a functional understanding of her condition and a mental ability and level of maturity consistent with the ability to comprehend the risks and benefits of a medical or treatment plan. She also needs to be able to give or withhold her permission from whatever care or treatment is offered. Many times it is not clear if someone is competent or not. Sometimes a psychological evaluation will need to be made to help determine the ability of a person to give consent for care. If a patient is considered incompetent, the health care team and the patient's family members or caregivers will need to determine who will serve as her legal guardian and make medical decisions for her. It is important to remember that the guardian needs to be available to give consent. Most public facilities, such as clinics, require that a written consent be signed at the initial visit to authorize permission to examine, diagnose, and treat a patient. Certainly, before any invasive procedure (e.g., biopsy, surgery) can be performed, it is necessary to obtain a signed informed consent, either from the patient if she's competent or from her legal guardian if she is not.

Many organizations, such Breast Health Access for Women with Disabilities (BHAWD), are aware of the necessity to increase the participation of women with disabilities in their own health care decisions. According to their vision statement, "BHAWD envisions a time when all women, including women with disabilities, will have the information and access to resources to obtain and advocate for their own health care and be seen as partners in their own health care" (BHAWD, March 2006).

Legal statutes govern reproductive health issues such as contraception, sterilization, and abortion. These rights vary from state to state and among institutions. It is best to know what applies locally. Resources for regional laws include local chapters of the American Civil Liberties Union, Planned Parenthood, the Alan Guttmacher Institute (http://www.agi-usa.org), or federally funded family planning services. The ethics committee of a hospital or health care institution may be called upon to settle complicated dilemmas involving reproductive health care for a woman with an intellectual or developmental disability who cannot consent for herself. Ethics committees are composed of representatives from various disciplines, such as nursing, medicine, psychiatry, social work, hospital administration, law, chaplaincy, and the community. If it appears that the legal guardian of a woman with an intellectual disability does not have the best interest of the woman in mind, a determination by an ethics committee may be warranted.

The laws governing a person's ability to provide meaningful and legal consent are more fully discussed in Chapter 9.

Lisa is 21 years old and has cerebral palsy, with a mild cognitive impairment. She uses a wheelchair to get around, and her ability to communicate is hampered by a speech impairment. With time and patience, however, Lisa is able to make her wishes known. Since the recent death of her mother, Lisa appears somewhat depressed. She now lives with her older sister, Jane, who has three young children. Lisa's relationship with her sister is strained. Lisa has become friendly with a man named Mike, the brother of a childhood friend, and Jane is concerned they will become sexually active. Jane made an appointment for Lisa at a local Planned Parenthood and wants Lisa to receive an injection of Depo-Provera (a long-acting contraceptive). Lisa had never been to this facility before and did not want to get this exam. While at the facility, Jane confronts the nurse practitioner, who is seeing Lisa for the first time, and says, "You have to give her the shot. I can't deal with her if she gets pregnant. I have more than enough on my plate taking care of her and my own kids."

The nurse practitioner ascertains that Lisa is competent to make her own health care decisions and determines that Jane is not her guardian. Lisa assures the nurse practitioner that she "wouldn't be stupid enough to get pregnant" and that her relationship with Mike is not a sexual one. She agrees to come back when and if she needs birth control. The nurse practitioner suggests a mental health referral for Lisa to address her feelings of sadness and to get help in improving her relationship with Jane. The nurse practitioner facilitates a conversation between Lisa and Jane to explain the current plan of care.

The above scenario describes a woman with an impaired ability to communicate, yet one who is competent. In other situations in which sexual activity is suspected and the woman is not competent, a guardian may decide a long-acting contraceptive, such as Depo-Provera, is warranted.

GYNECOLOGICAL EXAM

Having a pelvic exam can be stressful and embarrassing for many women. Stress and embarrassment can be heightened for a woman with an intellectual disability, especially if she has little understanding as to why an exam is needed, has had prior negative exam experiences, or has a history of victimization. Under these circumstances, an exam may even be terrifying. Compassion and commitment on the part of the health care professional to ease and calm the patient is critical. Sometimes, the assessment is best spread out over more than one visit. The first visit can be a time of introduction, history gathering, and educating the woman about the exam procedure. The second visit can be the exam itself.

Generally, a routine gynecologic evaluation includes an examination of the breasts and the teaching of breast exams in addition to a pelvic exam. The pelvic exam involves the use of a vaginal speculum to visualize inside the vagina and the cervix (the opening to the uterus). This is when a Pap test (screening for cervical cancer or precancerous changes) is obtained along with appropriate tests for various infections including sexually transmitted ones. Next, a bimanual exam (which involves the placement of one or two fingers inside the vagina while the other hand palpates over the lower abdomen) enables the clinician to feel the uterus and other pelvic organs. In addition, a rectal exam may be done. Most pelvic exams are done on a table with the woman lying on her back with her legs up in stirrups. A skilled provider will gently talk the woman through the exam, explaining what is happening as it proceeds and helping her to deep breathe and relax as best as possible. The provider also may use distraction techniques, such as telling stories or asking questions about the woman's interests. Most clients appreciate having a familiar support person accompany them throughout the visit.

The extent of the evaluation for a woman with an intellectual disability depends on a number of factors and may be approached in different ways. Obviously, teaching strategies for self-examination of breasts or the genitals will need to be individualized based on the type and level of disability, or may not be appropriate at all. BHAWD is an excellent resource for adaptive breast cancer detection and education approaches.

If a woman with an intellectual disability is unable to tolerate a speculum exam, a Pap test may be done "blindly" whereby a swab is inserted into the vagina to collect the specimen. The accuracy of the test is enhanced if the provider's finger is inserted first to guide the swab toward the cervix. Other specimens (for infections) can be collected similarly, and there now exist urine tests to check for common sexually transmitted infections. Some women are better able to accept a rectal exam than the bimanual exam. This still allows for some evaluation of the pelvic organs. Alternative positions may be needed for women with atypical anatomical structure, such as contracted limbs. A pelvic sonogram, which involves the placement of a probe onto the lower abdomen, can be a less threatening way to assess the uterus and ovaries, and may be ordered instead of or addition to the bimanual exam. Most women with mild to moderate intellectual disabilities are able to be examined by a sensitive provider using a combination of these techniques. When a patient is combative or not accepting of an evaluation that is deemed necessary, the gynecologic practitioner may recommend that the woman take a mild sedative or antianxiety medication just prior to the visit. Examination under anesthesia also remains an option for these circumstances.

The previously discussed issues of competency and guardianship come into play in situations in which the provider strongly recommends evaluation and/or treatment (e.g., for serious or life-threatening conditions) and the patient is unwilling.

Hope is 40 years old and is moderately cognitively disabled. She has never allowed anyone to do a gynecologic exam on her. For many years now, her periods have been infrequent and heavy. The last time she bled was 6 months ago. Her mother took her to the emergency room that day because she was bleeding very heavily and had become weak. Hope was found to be anemic and in need of a blood transfusion and as treatment to stop the bleeding. Hope had to have a gynecologic examination with Pap test, and a scraping of her uterus (D&C) performed under general anesthesia. No abnormal tissue in Hope's uterus was found; however, the provider did diagnose her with a hormonal imbalance. The provider prescribed treatment with a hormone medication to help prevent a recurrence of this circumstance.

A woman who has never allowed a gynecologic exam to be performed is sometimes in need of one during menopause to discover if postmenopausal symptoms require treatment.

Jenny has Down syndrome. She is 55 years old. She lives in a residential facility and has many friends and interests. Jenny is generally in good health. Lately, however, she has complained to her caretaker that her period has come back after 5 years with no periods. Jenny has never had sex and is unable to tolerate a thorough gynecologic exam. Her gynecologist expresses concern that the postmenopausal bleeding may be a warning sign for cancer and advises performing a biopsy of the uterus. It is not feasible, however, to perform this biopsy in the office. A meeting is called with Jenny's legal guardian, and Jenny's guardian consents to Jenny undergoing a gynecologic examination under anesthesia inclusive of the biopsy. During the examination, the gynecologist discovered and removed noncancerous polyps, and Jenny has had no further vaginal bleeding.

SEXUALLY TRANSMITTED INFECTIONS

STIs are considered a "hidden epidemic" in the United States in that they are often overlooked and misdiagnosed, resulting in serious consequences.

Women with intellectual disabilities have a greater than average incidence of sexual abuse (Morano, 2001). Abuse may go undetected for long periods of time, which can lead to untreated STIs with their health consequences as well as potential emotional and behavioral changes.

Yet, even women in consensual relationships get STIs. There are many different infections that can be contracted sexually. A routine OB-GYN examination does not always include testing for STIs. It is certainly appropriate, however, to ask for STI tests if there is even a remote possibility that one or more could be present. Some tests are performed on specimens obtained from the vagina or cervix while others are performed on the blood or urine. HIV testing can also be performed using swabs taken from the mouth. Many STIs have no symptoms, or symptoms may be subtle and easily missed.

Bacterial infections (e.g., gonorrhea, chlamydia) are treated and cured with antibiotics. Viral infections (e.g., herpes, HIV) may not be curable yet can be controlled through the use of medications. Also, some vaccines can prevent certain STIs. For example, Hepatitis A and B vaccines are available and recommended for anyone living in a group environment or at risk for an STI. A vaccine against strains of human papilloma virus (HPV), which are considered to be the cause of cervical cancer, is now available (Koutsky et al., 2002).

When a person is treated for an STI, it is always important to contact and treat their sexual partner(s) in order to decrease the chance of reinfection. Assisting the patient to incorporate behaviors to reduce her risk of getting another STI is essential. This can involve teaching her about her body and how infections are spread, identifying current or potential problems associated with the infection, finding alternate ways of meeting her needs for acceptance and love, and teaching the proper use of condoms to help prevent contracting infections in the future.

Kerry is in her late 20s and has a mild cognitive impairment; however, she is considered competent to consent for care. Kerry has suffered multiple traumas in her short life. For example, several years ago, she was badly burned in a house fire during which her best friend was killed. In addition, her mother died recently, and she is now living with a cousin and she has an intensive outpatient mental health team. During a gynecologic visit, which was a follow-up visit due to abnormal Pap test results 6 months earlier, Kerry disclosed to the GYN nurse practitioner that she had become sexually active and has not used protection. Kerry's exam revealed significant inflammation of the vaginal walls with a malodorous vaginal discharge. Testing found infection with trichomoniasis, which is an STI treatable with antibiotics and often co-exists with other STIs. Kerry's Pap test was deferred until the infection was cleared, and instead, an STI workup was done. The nurse practitioner educated Kerry about the nature of trichomoniasis infection and explained to her that her sexual partner needed treatment as well and that she is at risk for other STIs. Pregnancy risk counseling was also initiated, and, with Kerry's permission, her social worker was notified of the situation.

Kerry returned 1 month later and stated that she had not had sex since the last visit. During this visit, the Pap smear was again abnormal, showing precancerous changes that require further investigation. This is likely due to co-infection with HPV.

There is still more to Kerry's story and presenting medical issues.

Kerry has not had regular periods since the fire. For the first year, she did not bleed at all. Since then, her periods have been very infrequent. A workup inclusive of blood hormone studies has concluded this is due to her medications and obesity. She takes two antidepressants, which can cause hormonal changes and lack of periods. Obesity, which can be a side effect of psychiatric drugs, is also associated with menstrual irregularities. Treatment is important to protect her from developing cancer of the lining of the uterus later in life, as both obesity and skipping periods are risk factors for uterine cancer.

CONTRACEPTION OPTIONS

There are various contraception options available, and many factors need to be considered to determine which option is best suited for each individual. Some methods are controlled by the individual and others are more closely monitored by a provider. Over recent years, much effort has been placed on developing new methods with ease of use in mind.

Hormonal methods of contraception now include the birth control pill, patch, and shot, in addition to the vaginal ring. These are all prescribed by and then monitored by a health care provider and are highly effective at preventing pregnancy when used correctly. The pill needs to be taken at the same time each day, whereas the patch is worn on the skin for a week and then removed and replaced by a new patch. Each cycle consists of wearing a new patch weekly for 3 weeks and one "patch-free" week when bleeding is expected. The Depo-Provera shot is given once every 3 months. The vaginal ring is inserted in the vagina and left inside for 3 weeks, at which point it is removed, discarded, and left out for one week before a new ring is inserted and a new cycle begins. An "under-the-skin" implant consisting of one hormone-bearing rod has been approved by the Food & Drug Administration and provides effective contraception for up to 3 years (Peck 2006, July 19).

The shot and implant contain progesterone alone, while the other methods contain a combination of estrogen and progesterone (female hormones). It is important to realize that the progesterone-only methods versus the combined (estrogen and progesterone) ones have different side effects, risks, and benefits. For example, estrogen-containing methods may increase the risk of developing a blood clot, especially for certain women. (This reinforces the importance of providing an accurate medical and family history.) And while progesterone alone is likely to cause irregular or no periods, most women who use a combined method generally have predictable, shorter periods with less cramping. There is even a new way of prescribing combination pills that leads to only four periods per year. Hormonal methods can cause or aggravate mood swings for some, may cause headaches for others, may increase the risk of seizures in women with an underlying seizure disorder, and/or may interact with other prescribed medications. Conversely, they may reduce the chance of developing anemia, osteoporosis, pelvic infections, cysts, and even cancer of the ovaries and uterus.

The gynecologic health care provider should be an excellent resource in sorting out the nuances of the different hormonal options and coming up with an individualized plan that is best suited to each woman. Consideration needs to be given to the woman's ability to comply with the method instructions and what support system she has to assist her. Can she be relied upon to take a pill daily or will it be administered to her? Would it be easier to get a shot once every 3 months?

Barrier methods of birth control include condoms, diaphragms, and vaginal spermicides (e.g., foams, creams, suppositories, the sponge). Even when used correctly, barrier methods of contraception are significantly less effective in preventing pregnancy than hormonal methods. They require good hand coordination and dexterity as well as a motivated, capable couple to use properly. Local irritation, difficulty with insertion and removal, and unwanted pregnancy are all potential side effects. Vaginal spermicides may actually increase a woman's risk of becoming infected with HIV if irritation of the vagina is present and she is exposed to the virus.

Still, condoms remain a highly effective means of protection against STIs for sexually active individuals (Cates & Stone, 1992; Centers for Disease Control [CDC], 1998). Condoms are recommended in addition to hormonal methods in circumstances in which there is potential for acquisition of STIs, and both women and men should be educated in their use. "The condom is recognized as a highly effective barrier against HIV infection" (CDC, 2004).

Intrauterine devices (IUDs) are long-term methods of contraception, which allow 5 to 10 years of highly effective, reversible birth control. IUDs available in the U.S. are made of plastic, along with either copper or progesterone, and are placed within the uterus during a vaginal exam by the health care provider. There was a poorly designed IUD, the Dalkon Shield, used in the 1970s, which caused dangerous problems for many women, including serious infections of the pelvis that led to hysterectomies for some and even deaths for others (Tatum, Schmidt, Philips, McCarty, & O'Leary, 1975). The Dalkon Shield was taken off the market many years ago, and the IUDs used currently in the United States for appropriately screened women are much safer. In addition, the likelihood of becoming pregnant when wearing an IUD is about the same as for surgical steriliazation.

Although there may still be risks associated with IUDs, their safety and effectiveness have been well-documented for appropriately screened women (ACOG, January 2005). There are no systemic side effects or potential drug interactions associated with copper IUD, and only minimal hormone-related effects noted with progesterone IUD. Potential problems associated with either IUD include expulsion of device, pelvic infection which primarily occurs soon after insertion or in association with an STI, pelvic pain, menstrual changes, and a very small risk of perforation of the uterus. Some women experience increased vaginal bleeding and menstrual cramping when a copper IUD is inserted, and this can be cause for removal of the device from the woman. Conversely, the progesterone IUD may be used as a treatment to control heavy bleeding. While unlikely, hormone related effects such as headache, nausea, breast tenderness, and depression may occur in women who have the progesterone IUD. If a woman with an IUD becomes infected with an STI, the STI can progress quickly and lead to severe infection, chronic pain, infertility, and even the need for a hysterectomy. As such, use of IUDs is generally limited to married women in monogamous relationships. Women who may not be able to verbalize symptoms of pain or infection should never be given an IUD.

SURGICAL STERILIZATION

Surgical sterilization via removal or destruction of the fallopian tubes (tubal ligation) is the most effective method of contraception, with a failure rate of 13 pregnancies per 1000 procedures over 5 years (ACOG, September 2003). Tubal ligation is considered permanent and irreversible; therefore, it should never be performed without careful consideration and counseling. Most women can have a tubal ligation performed under general anesthesia in a hospital operating room through a small incision at the navel and are able to go home the same day. Recovery is generally quick with abdominal discomfort for a few days and a low chance of infection. As a surgical procedure, there still exists the unlikely potential of unforeseen complications, which can result in a longer hospital stay or a more extensive surgery. Sometimes a larger, yet still small, lower abdominal incision is needed in order to access the fallopian tubes. A hysterectomy is another form of sterilization, which also stops menstruation; however, it is not considered appropriate for most women due to the higher risk of surgery-related complications.

For women with intellectual disabilities, sterilization brings up historical, legal, and ethical issues. In the days when people with disabilities were hidden from society, sterilization was often forced upon women with disabilities to prevent them from reproducing and further "tainting" society as a whole. In 1942, the Supreme Court determined that this practice of mandatory sterilization of people with disabilities was unconstitutional (Baylor College of Medicine, 1997). State statutes regarding this issue vary. Some states prohibit sterilization of a person with a mental disability entirely, while others do allow the procedure with caveats. A key issue is whether the person is competent to consent to the surgery. For example, in Texas, only the woman herself can give informed consent to be sterilized. If she is incapable of consenting, the procedure cannot be performed. This may not be overturned by legal guardians or even a court (Advocacy, Inc., n.d.). In Oregon, a petition must be filed with the state court to determine if sterilization is in the best interest of the woman with the disability who cannot consent for herself (Oregon Advocacy Center, 2002). In other places, a team of medical and nonmedical individuals, such as an ethics committee, will be called upon to make this decision.

SEX EDUCATION

Sex education is a process that starts in childhood and is a lifelong course of study. Unfortunately, many families and caregivers feel ill equipped and embarrassed to deal with the subject of sex. Individuals with developmental disabilities typically need special assistance and unique materials and teaching strategies for sex education to be truly meaningful and effective. This education needs to go beyond simply knowing about reproductive anatomy and physiological processes and functions. It needs to include positive relationship skills, assertiveness training, decision making practice, self-protection skills that will enhance personal safety, social skills that support appropriate behaviors and allow the expression of affection, love and intimacy, and supervised as well as more independent opportunities to interact with people to whom they are attracted. At the end of this chapter there are additional resources that may be helpful to the reader.

Many commercially prepared special educational materials are useful for teaching about sexual health, but, education may also include experiences that are not so formal:

- A "readiness training" visit to a family planning clinic or physician's office when it is not in use can be an excellent learning opportunity. The visit offers a chance to see what the atmosphere is like and who works there.

- A classroom teacher or school or guest nurse can show young women a speculum and allow the woman to handle it as a way of knowing what is happening to her.

- Viewing library photographs and mainstream videos that are available for rent or purchase can make abstract ideas of pregnancy and birth less glorified and very, very real.

- A guest speaker who knows personally about HIV/AIDS or other STIs can create a powerful and unforgettable learning experience.

- Collecting an assortment of birth control materials that women and men could handle in a leisurely way, outside of a medical environment, is a fascinating and enlightening way to spend an hour or two with a small group of adults.

There are chances for education available frequently, if caregivers and teachers choose to use them. The creative educational strategies and unique learning techniques and materials addressed in this and many of the previous chapters of this book make sex education possible for men and women with intellectual limitations. Ideally, educational programs will become more widespread in their use and availability to help women with disabilities, their partners, and their support systems negotiate this very important aspect of a women's sexual health (and men's too!).

PREGNANCY

When a woman with an intellectual disability becomes pregnant, as for any pregnant woman, a multitude of decisions need to be made. For a woman with an intellectual disability, the issues related to her disability usually have a significant impact on this process. Once the pregnancy is confirmed and the health situation of the pregnant woman and fetus is safeguarded, choices related to parenting, foster care, adoption, or ter-mination must be addressed. The sea of complex legal, ethical, social, and moral considerations in making the decision to continue or termi-nate the pregnancy must be navigated cautiously and with skill to ensure that the woman knows and understands the choice she is making, whichever one it may be, and the long-term implications of that choice. Social workers and psychologists as well as medical personnel all need to participate in providing information about the risks and benefits of all choices and verify whether the woman is able to make this decision with support or whether this decision will be made for her by her guardian. It is important that at least the decision to either continue the pregnan-cy or terminate it be made as early in the pregnancy as possible, as it becomes more difficult to terminate a pregnancy after 12 weeks have passed. So while other decisions can be delayed, termination decisions should not be delayed.

If a woman or her guardian chooses to terminate the pregnancy, an abortion should be performed in accordance with the law. These laws vary from state to state. Adequate plans for counseling of the woman should be made with a person skilled in working with individuals who have an intellectual disability.

If the choice is made to continue the pregnancy, ongoing discus-sion about the woman's or couple's plans for the future of the baby needs to be had, and ongoing support for a healthy prenatal life style that is free of alcohol, illegal drugs and harmful prescription drug inter-actions must be begun as soon as possible.

When a female patient with an intellectual or developmental dis-ability seeks to continue her pregnancy, the first order of business is med-ical care. Locating an appropriate medical facility for prenatal care and delivery is of great importance. Many patients with a developmental dis-ability can have inadequate preventive medical services; there may well be a multitude of concurrent medical problems, some undiagnosed or untreated. Social issues and financial limitations, compounded with other ongoing medical conditions, can make pregnancy a more compli-cated process for some women with disabilities. In selecting a pregnancy-monitoring locale, it is often beneficial to choose a medical facility that has ongoing access to multiple disciplines and medical sub specialists. A social worker can arrange for home health care assistance, financial assis-tance, coordinate registration with Medicaid, if necessary, and/or other government programs, and assist with any difficult home living situa-tions. A nutritionist can ensure that the patient receives all the necessary nutritional requirements for both mother and baby, as well as provide guidance when pregnancies are complicated by diabetes, obesity, inade-quate weight gain, or other nutrition related problems not yet discovered. The patient may have other medical problems that can have an impact on both mother and baby or the pregnancy. Easy access to medical providers in such fields as internal medicine, surgery, neurology, psychiatry, endocrinology, genetic counseling, or others may be needed.

If a patient plans to put the newborn infant up for adoption, the appropriate agencies should be contacted as soon as possible in order to make the necessary legal and financial arrangements. If a mother-to-be or couple plans to assume a parental role, issues of patient competency and the ultimate custody of the newborn infant should be addressed as early in the pregnancy as possible. This issue can be resolved in discussions among the patient, immediate family members, other guardians or caregivers, and medical center staff. Early involvement of hospital administration and nursery department supervisory staff will insure that after birth there is no delay in the discharge home of mother and baby due to legal or administrative problems. Once again, a large facility with access to social workers, legal counsel, and experienced administration will facilitate easy navigation through these potential difficulties.

It is no longer an automatic decision that a child is removed from the custody of his or her parents, if one or both of the parents has an intellectual disability. Parenting classes, in-home child care training, and ongoing social, emotional, and psychological support can teach effective and safe parenting skills to these new parents. Often, involved grandparents are delighted to play an important guiding role and are themselves revitalized by committing to their son or daughter to assist on an ongoing basis to help raise the new addition to the family.

The complexity of the mother's disability, accompanying medical and social problems, and even the patient's access to transportation, can make pregnancy complicated. It is often most practical and safe for the patient to receive prenatal care and deliver at a university medical center or other integrated public health facility.

Pregnancy care typically involves approximately fifteen prenatal visits with a health care provider. More visits may be necessary in pregnancies with medical complications. The health care provider will determine the need for additional visits. It is absolutely vital that the patient or accompanying guardian or caregiver be prepared at each visit to discuss any and all medical problems and symptoms. The effects of seemingly minor complaints or symptoms may be greatly magnified in pregnancy, where any complaint can impact directly on a developing fetus. In addition, the health care provider may be offering important advice and instructions such as what foods and medications are safe in pregnancy, and what symptoms may indicate a problem requiring immediate medical intervention. Problems such as preterm labor, premature rupture of membranes, toxemia, and placental abruption are emergencies and necessitate immediate evaluation and treatment. The patient and any guardian or caregiver will need to be aware of the early signs of these problems.

The expectant woman with an intellectual disability needs comprehensive information about what to expect during pregnancy and birth in a language and a format that is consistent with how she learns and understands new information. She should learn about the need for her own health care and nutrition and the impact of her weight on the pregnancy and child to come. The woman must be informed of and guided through the biological changes during each stage of pregnancy, the difference in her center of balance, what labor is, how to prepare for labor by taking birth classes and hospital tours, and what pain relief and anesthesia choices are available to her.

During the actual labor and delivery, many hospitals allow the presence of only one spouse, partner, or other supporting individual. The patient with an intellectual disability may require the presence of a number of family members and other supporters in order to assist with the physical and emotional challenges of labor. These arrangements should be made with the patient, her advocates, caregivers or family members, the labor and delivery staff, and perhaps a social worker or advocate in advance of the delivery date.

Today, labor and delivery need not be an impossibly painful process. Numerous techniques and medical interventions are available to lessen the discomfort:

- Lamaze and other relaxation techniques
- Various types of pain medications including narcotics
- Anesthesia, usually epidural (via the spine) or general (much less common)

The patient's knowledge and familiarity with the hospital, and the information about what to expect from pregnancy, labor and delivery, all serve to alleviate to some degree the patient's anxiety about this wondrous, but sometimes frightening, experience.

SUMMARY

It is clear that although the information and issues of OB-GYN care for women with intellectual or developmental disabilities are identical in many ways to those of other women, the manner in which the information is conveyed, the way that understanding is assured, and the way that support is given can differ markedly. It cannot be overemphasized that with more complete and accurate historical information, the OB-GYN health care provider can ensure better care. This often places the guardian or caregiver in a unique role that simultaneously asks for more involvement while still fostering the woman's independence. Guardianship, level of competency, and state laws complicate issues of reproductive health care for patients with intellectual disabilities.

REFERENCES

American College of Obstetricians and Gynecologists. (2003, April.). Clinical management guidelines for the obstetrician-gynecologist: Breast cancer screening. *Practice Bulletin #42*. Washington, DC: Author.

American College of Obstetricians and Gynecologists. (2003, August). Clinical management guidelines for the obstetrician-gynecologist: Cervical cytology screening. *Practice Bulletin #45*. Washington, DC: Author.

American College of Obstetricians and Gynecologists. (2003, September). Risks and benefits of sterilization. *Practice Bulletin #46*. Washington, DC: Author.

American College of Obstetricians and Gynecologists. (2005, January). Intrauterine device. *Practice Bulletin #59*. Washington, DC: Author.

Association of State and Territorial Health Officials. (2003, May). *Access to preventative health care services for women with disabilities*. Fact Sheet. Washington, DC: Author.

Advocacy, Inc. (n.d.). *Sterilization of persons with mental disabilities: Advocating the legal rights of Texans with disabilities*. Retrieved July 11, 2006, from http://advocacyinc.org/CS7_text.htm

Baylor College of Medicine (1997, September). Reproductive healthcare for the mentally handicapped. *The Contraception Report, 8*(4). Retrieved July 11, 2006, from http://www.contraceptiononline.org/contrareport/article01.cfm?art=31

Breast Health Access for Women with Disabilities. Vision statement. Retrieved March 26, 2006, from http://www.bhawd.org/sitefiles/vision.html

Cates, W. & Stone, K.M. (1992). Family planning, sexually transmitted diseases, and contraceptive choice: A literature update—Part I. *Family Planning Perspectives, 24*(2), 75–84.

Centers for Disease Control and Prevention. (1998). 1998 guidelines for the treatment of sexually transmitted diseases. *Morbidity and Mortality Weekly Report, 47*, 1–116.

Centers for Disease Control and Prevention. (2004). *Fact sheet for public health personnel: Male latex condoms and sexually transmitted diseases*. Retrieved June 7, 2004, from http://www.cdc.gov/nchstp/od/latex.htm

Koutsky, L.A., Ault, K.A., Wheeler, C.M., Brown, D.R., Bar, E., Alvarez, F.B., et al. (2002). A controlled trial of human papillomavirus type 16 vaccine. *New England Journal of Medicine, 347*(21), 1645–1651.

Oregon Advocacy Center. (2002). *A guide to Oregon's sterilization law*. Retrieved July 10, 2006, from http://www.oradvocacy.org/pubs/sterilization.htm

Morano, J.P. (2001). Sexual abuse of the mentally retarded patient: Medical and legal analysis for the primary care physician. *Primary Care Companion, Journal of Clinical Psychiatry, 3*(3), 126–135.

Peck, P. (2006, July 19). FDA approves matchstick-sized contraceptive implant. *MedPage Today*. Retrieved July 19, 2006, from http://www.medpagetoday.com /ProductAlert/DevicesandVaccines/tb/3748

Tatum, H.J., Schmidt, F.H., Phillips, D., McCarty, M., & O'Leary, W.M. (1975). The Dalkon Shield controversy: Structural and bacteriological studies of IUD tails. *Journal of the American Medical Association, 231*(17), 711–717.

Tezzoni, L.I., McCarthy, E.P., Davis, R.B., Harris-David, L., & O'Day, B. (2001). Use of screening & preventative services among women with disabilities. *American Journal of Medical Quality, 16*(4), 135–144.

U.S. Department of Health & Human Services. (2000). *Healthy people 2010: Understanding & improving health.* Washington, DC: U.S. Government Printing Office.

Welner, S.A. (1999). *Provider's guide for the care of women with physical disabilities and chronic medical conditions.* University of Maryland, Baltimore: North Carolina Office on Disability & Health.

RESOURCES

American Association of Mental Retardation
http://www.aamr.org

American Civil Liberties Union
http://www.aclu.org/disability/index.html

The Arc
http://www.thearc.org

Center for Disease Control Office of Women's Health
http://www.cdc.gov/women/az/disabil.htm

Center for Health Rights
http://www.healthcarerrights.org

Center for Research on Women with Disabilities at Texas Baylor College of Medicine
http://www.bcm.edu/crowd/index.cfm

National Down Syndrome Congress
http://www.ndsccenter.org

Planned Parenthood Federation of America
http://www.PPFA.org

12

Helping Individuals Recover from Sexual Abuse

One Therapist's Model

Marklyn P. Champagne

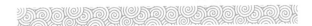

"It cannot be repeated too often that persons with MR/DD may be misperceived to be less disturbed by traumatic events because they are misperceived as less aware." Andrew S. Levitas, M. D., and Stephen F. Gilson, Ph.D., 2001.

The following case illustration demonstrates the complexity of thoughts, feelings, and actions experienced by Lanie, a 29-year-old woman with a moderate intellectual disability living in a residential home, after repeated sexual assaults perpetrated by a trusted male staff member. After disclosing the simple statement "He touched me," Lanie was referred for assessment and treatment of posttraumatic stress disorder (PTSD).

Imagine that he says to you, "It's all your fault, you're so pretty!" He then smothers you with kisses smelling of his cigarette and coffee breath. Imagine that he commands you, "Go to the back of the van. Take down your pants!" Then, he rapes you with suntan lotion as a lubricant. Imagine that he then says to you, "If you tell anyone, I will lose my job and my wife will divorce me."

Imagine that he shoves your face into the rough cloth and the stink of the van carpet; imagine the pain of an anal rape; imagine the loneliness of being overpowered. Imagine the responsibility for believing you are the cause of this rape. Imagine the responsibility of believing that your disclosure will cause suffering to his wife and family because he will lose his job and they will leave him.

Imagine the fear and anticipation for 12 long months that any day this male staff member will drive you to your job and any day may decide to rape you again. Imagine the pain and humiliation each time it happens. Imagine feeling dirty and bad.

Lanie struggled to find the words to describe these heinous acts: "Down there?" "Behind?" "Lotion for the beach?" "His thing?"

Imagine the nightmares, isolation, and the feeling that people will look at you and know: It was your fault. Imagine the panic when the nurse asks to speak with you alone. The nurse announces, "Ed is in jail." You think, "I'm in big trouble now." The nurse continues, "He did something very bad, he touched other women in their private parts." You think jumbled thoughts: Other women? Who? Not just me? What are private parts? Will I lose my job? Will he lose his job? What will my mom and dad do?

"Yeah, he touched me." Terror. The nurse continues, "It's not your fault." More jumbled thoughts: "What will happen to me now?"

WHAT IS SEXUAL ASSAULT?

The international public health perspective defines *sexual violence* as "any sexual act, attempt to obtain a sexual act, unwanted sexual comments or advances . . . against a person's sexuality using coercion, by any person regardless of their relationship to the victim in any setting, including, but not limited to home and work"(Kilpatrick, 2004, pp. 1214–1215). *Coercion* is defined as "including physical force, psychological intimidation. . . . or taking advantage of an individual who is unable to give consent because they are . . . mentally incapable of understanding the situation" (Kilpatrick, 2004, p. 1215).

For purposes of this chapter, the terms *sexual assault* and *abuse* are used to describe the acts of violence against a non-consenting person. These acts are committed for the gratification of the perpetrator and may involve a range of offenses including, but not limited to, using sexually explicit language and pornography, touching sexual body parts, and/or oral, vaginal, and anal rape (Nettlebeck, Wilson, Potter, & Perry, 2000). Each state has its own specific legal definition of sexual assault. (For specific information about a specific state, readers should contact the State Attorney General's office from that state.)

VULNERABILITY

Nationally, abuse statistics are kept for the general population but do not specify the number of assaults against people with intellectual disabilities. In the general population, 20% of females and 5%–10% of males are suspected of being victims of sexual abuse annually (Reynolds, 1997). Studies conducted specifically among people with intellectual disabilities indicated that they are 4 to 10 times more likely to be victimized than individuals in the general population (Sobsey, 1994). In one study, 83% of the women with intellectual disabilities surveyed reported to have been sexually abused at some point in their lives, and of those, 50% reported to have been sexually assaulted 10 or more times (Petersilia, Foote, & Crowell, 2001). The literature indicates that the numbers of males with intellectual disabilities who report being victims of sexual assault may be much higher than reported. When men disclose sexual assault, they report "shock, humiliation, embarrassment, and behavioral changes" that persist for years, and men are said to experience more "anger, irritability, conflicting sexual orientation, loss of self-respect, and sexual dysfunction similar to female rape victims" (Stermac & Del Bove, 2004, p. 902).

When sexual assault is understood as an issue of power and control, the particular vulnerability of the person with an intellectual disability becomes more apparent. The disparity of cognitive ability between perpetrators of typical intelligence and individuals with intellectual disabilities make trickery and coercion more likely to occur. There are perpetrators who intend power in the relationship rather than violence against another. Power "include[s] threats, intimidation, neglect, and acts of omission" (Kilpatrick, 2004, p. 1214). Perpetrators often choose their victims because of the victim's intellectual disability, figuring that detection is unlikely. Since victims with intellectual disabilities often have limited ability to recognize and report sexual abuse, may lack the skills to get help, are likely to be overly compliant, have little decision making power of their own, and are frequently in positions of dependency, perpetrators can maintain access to their victims for long periods of time (Sobsey, 1994).

As a group, individuals with intellectual disabilities are more passive, more easily dominated, and frequently are taught to act to please authority figures. They often have impaired logical thinking and more limited problem-solving abilities, especially when compounded by limits in reasoning abilities, foresight, and strategic thinking (Wall, Krupp, & Guilmette, 2003). Individuals with intellectual disabilities also may lack communication skills because of limited vocabulary, poor articulation, and difficulty with syntax. All of these factors contribute to the diminished ability of a person with an intellectual disability to report abuse (Wall et al., 2003). In addition, individuals with intellectual disabilities are often unable to anticipate danger or do not have the awareness, language, and assertiveness skills to try to protect themselves at appropriate times (Petersilia et al., 2001).

HOW IS SEXUAL ABUSE DISCLOSED OR DISCOVERED?

Sexual abuse is often not disclosed until the victim feels safe, which may be months or years after the abuse has occurred, particularly if the individual continues to fear threats by the assailant. Sometimes, however, the victim does file a report and is not believed. Many times, discovery occurs only after manifestations of maladaptive behaviors, rather than a verbal recounting of the abuse. Sexualized behaviors, sexual aggression, forced exposure of others' genitals, compulsive masturbation, and the simulation of intercourse with dolls, peers, or animals are important signs that abuse may have occurred (Johnson, 1999). Other less serious, but nevertheless important, signs of abuse include drastic changes in appetite, behavior, and/or personality; anxiety, irritability, and constant inattentiveness; and anger, threats to do harm, and nightmares (Johnson, 1999).

> Lanie had been successfully employed for many years as a preparation chef. After a few months, however, she began to demonstrate a reluctance to go to work. She cut her hand several times with a knife, seemingly by accident, and she fell, hurting her ankle. Lanie uncharacteristically also began seeking the nurse's attention for vague body complaints.

Indirect discovery of sexual abuse can also occur with pregnancy, infection with a sexually transmitted disease, and/or injuries such as vaginal or anal tearing. A rape exam is best performed within 72 hours of an assault for both treatment and evidence collection. However, even if a rape exam is not completed within that period, a medical exam is still necessary to document and, most importantly, treat any concomitant physical problems.

If sexual abuse has occurred over an extended period of time, a person with an intellectual disability may not be able to provide an accurate chronology of the abuse. He or she may give snippets of information, out of order, and seemingly unrelated. Although this inconsistency is not detrimental to treatment, it does make the disclosure less credible in the legal system and can make prosecution less likely.

INTAKE: BEGINNING ASSESSMENT, DIAGNOSIS, AND TREATMENT

Often when an individual without intellectual disabilities has been sexually assaulted, he or she can seek treatment from a skilled therapist.

The individual has the capacity to verbally express the trauma and benefit from the therapist's resources through traditional talk therapy. For an individual with an intellectual disability, many supports can be needed to gain access to therapy. Help finding a suitable therapist skilled in working with individuals with intellectual disabilities and trauma, transportation and therapeutic support outside of the therapist's hourly session can be necessary.

It is most often a trusted, helping individual that identifies and calls a skilled therapist to set up an appointment for intake, the first step toward treatment for individuals suffering from the effects of sexual abuse. A therapist initiates intake by conducting a telephone interview for information about the victim, including current status regarding the alleged incidents, the most pressing symptoms and, current coping mechanisms, supports, and other pertinent information. After this initial interview, the therapist encourages a trusted staff or family member to attend at least part of the therapy sessions with the person. The therapist would honor the individual's requests for or against having a supportive person attend the therapeutic sessions and in selecting who would be helpful during the day-to-day healing process (which can sometimes involve 24-hour supports). Depending on the individual's desire, the support person may attend all or part of the session but is typically given an opportunity to engage in the last 15 minutes to help plan the follow-up assignments for coping throughout the week. This alliance with a support person is necessary in order to remind and encourage the individual to employ treatment strategies on an ongoing basis, to practice and refine coping strategies, and to lend encouragement and support.

Many times, the therapist will encourage the support person to speak about the therapeutic process and his or her own personal trust of the therapist (if one is established) to hasten the therapeutic alliance and create a triad of healing individuals.

> At intake, Lanie was well dressed and wore her hair stylishly cut. She was personable, and, while she would respond in short, nondescriptive sentences to specific questions, she had difficulty with expressive language and was reluctant to offer information about her sexual abuse. Lanie's insight was limited and in part indicative of her enduring perception that she was "in trouble" for the abuse. She seemed unsure about the nature of the counseling visit.

The individual who has suffered sexual abuse acts as the most significant self-healer and director of the therapeutic process. To quickly facilitate building trust and safety at the intake appointment, the therapist greets the individual and the support person. The therapist asks if the individual wishes that the support person be included for any part of the session. This diminishes the individual's fear of being alone with the therapist (as the person was alone with the perpetrator), increases trust, and also immediately clarifies that the individual will be given choices and will not be forced to participate in uncomfortable situations. If the individual invites the support person for the first part of the session, that can facilitate building trust and gathering information and begins the process of creating a triad of healers including the individual, the support person, and the therapist. A release of information is always required.

The intake process begins with an explanation of the counseling process, which is simplified by saying, "The work here is to make sure you are happy, feeling good, and doing well at home and work." The therapist inquires about date of birth, address, and other biographical information for purposes of evaluating cognitive and language abilities and to observe the person's overall verbal, cognitive, and mental status. Such questions can also offer power and a sense of capability to the individual.

The therapist also explains issues of confidentiality in language that the person understands. The therapist may begin the confidentiality conversation by saying, "What is said in this room stays in this room, but there will be times when information has to be shared to keep you and others safe." The therapist informs the person of his or her duty to report abuse not already disclosed and to report threats of self-injury or threats to cause harm to another based on national laws (*Tarasoff v. University of California,* 1976). Each state has its own laws and definitions of protected persons and what constitutes abuse. Therapists must be familiar with the rules governing their states. (Check individual state laws for comprehensive information.)

The therapist uses language that is simple and direct to ascertain the individual's understanding by asking the individual to repeat what the therapist has said in the individual's own words. If the issues of the work of therapy and confidentiality are not clear to the individual, the therapist can use even more simplified language and slowly repeat each topic until there is evidence that the person has a sense of the therapeutic work and the limits of confidentiality.

To reassure the person of the therapist's role and to facilitate disclosure, the therapist might say, "People who feel unhappy, hurt, scared, not quite like they did before, or who have had bad touches come here every day. Your support person told me a little bit about what happened to you." The therapist can then show the PTSD Assessment and Treatment Model (see Figure 12.1) to the individual. Most individuals feel

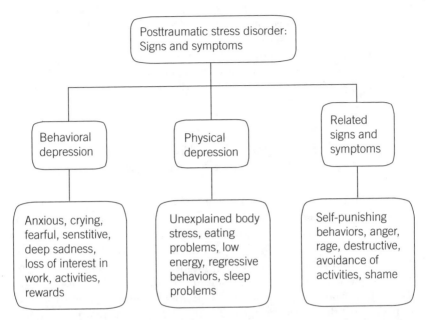

Figure 12.1. Posttraumatic stress disorder assessment and treatment model. (Adapted from Reiss, S. [1988]. *Reiss screen for maladaptive behavior.* Worthington, OH: IDS Publishing Corporation.)

very alone in their abuse experience. Therefore, telling them that other people have been hurt and can feel better also begins to de-stigmatize the individual's experience and increase the individual's confidence in his or her own ability to begin the healing process.

After establishing initial trust, the therapist's first goal is to help the person express the aspects of abuse that are most distressing at the time. This might include disclosing some aspects of the abuse or the symptoms that are the aftermath of abuse. The therapist should reassure the individual that he or she has heard these aspects and/or symptoms before from others who have been sexually abused. Because reports of abuse may not occur in chronological order, this approach seems to work best to meet individuals' needs as they arise. The therapist must note the assessment of the symptoms—where and when they occurred and the severity. The methods for soothing the individual and the strategies for achieving specific treatment goals and objectives must be developed in partnership with the individual, the support person, if he or she is invited, and the therapist.

The therapist should also perform a comparison between the individual's highest level of function prior to the assault and the individual's current level of functioning in areas such as biological, psychological, and social status. (American Psychiatric Association, 2000)

> Even though Lanie had minimal reading skills, she was presented with a written and illustrated paper simply titled PTSD and was informed of what the writing meant through referring to the pictures that supported the written language.

HOW A PERSON IS ASSESSED FOR DIAGNOSIS AND LATER TREATMENT

Androgynous drawings can aid communication between a therapist and an individual undergoing treatment for sexual abuse. Pictorial support assists the individual in communicating with the therapist, especially if the individual has diminished expressive skills. The individual can then accurately report symptoms without language being so great a barrier.

The drawings used should relate to the aftermath of abuse and the sense of imbalance and depression that are common after abusive experiences. The drawings should indicate a correlation of those feelings with the abuse experience, which can make disclosure easier. This step provides an explanation of feelings and behaviors and acknowledges that other people have experienced similar abuse and the person is not alone in the healing process.

The assessment and treatment model shown in Figure 12.2 represents imbalance and the differing positions of balance by labeling them Flight, Numb, and Fight and then associating them with specific thoughts, feelings, and behaviors. This oversimplified description minimizes the use of language to describe and report symptoms and teaches the individual a more concrete way of expressing or denying symptoms of distress. By describing and modeling the swaying of the seats through up and down gestures (i.e., the loss of balance and control) PTSD symptoms can be described and communicated. The therapist can visually demonstrate that trauma symptoms are not static and can describe and illustrate the thoughts, feelings, and behaviors a person may experience in all three of the balance positions. For example, at one moment, the individual may feel angry and irritable (Fight) and the next moment feel overwhelmed with memories and emotion (Flight) or feel detached (Numb) to keep thoughts at bay. All three states interfere with daily activities and interrupt normal activities.

The reexperiencing of intrusive memories (Flight) exists when the traumatic event replays in the person's mind as if the event were reoccurring again (e.g., flashbacks). Some people describe this as a movie

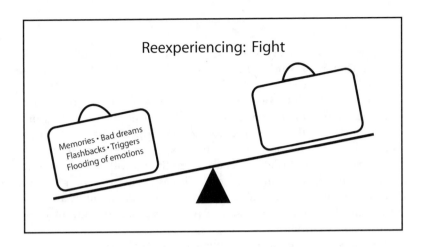

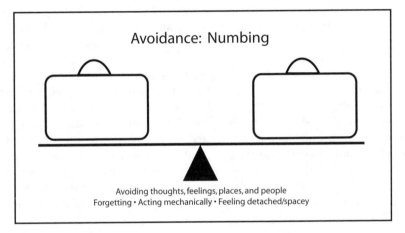

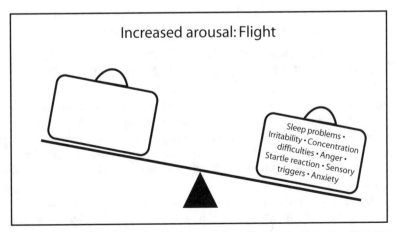

Figure 12.2. Posttraumatic stress disorder flight/numb/fight. Figure designed by Jason Wertheimer.

playing over and over again in the mind, or as a series of still photographs. This may produce a highly aroused and terrified state, and the individual may appear to be flooded with emotions.

Avoidance (Numb) occurs when the person tries to stop remembering the abuse and actively avoids people, places, or things that bring back memories. In this state, the person may appear glassy eyed, forgetful, detached, and mechanical, and may express no enjoyment.

Increased arousal (Fight) occurs when the individual feels as if trauma may occur again at any moment. This is a state of hyper vigilance when the person may experience sleep problems, irritability, anger, difficulty concentrating, intense startle reactions, anxiety, and an overresponsiveness to stimuli.

The person may experience any of these PTSD symptoms individually or simultaneously. Obviously, symptoms are not as simple or clearcut as the table presents. The symptoms can vary in intensity and severity and can vacillate quickly. The individual may feel as if the trauma is happening in the present.

Sensory stimuli such as touch, taste, smell, sound, and images that launch movement between these three states are called *triggers*. Triggers are defined as those sensory stimuli, memories, or feelings that "set off" a memory of an abusive situation. Usually, the therapist has to first educate the individual about this concept and then help the individual explore and discover the triggers that may come at unforeseen times and cause emotional distress. When triggering experiences can be found through assessment, discovery actions can then be taken to diminish exposure to the triggers and to develop tools to respond to them differently.

ADJUNCT THERAPY FOR PTSD AND THE ASSOCIATION WITH OTHER MENTAL ILLNESSES: WHAT IS THE THERAPIST'S ROLE AFTER ASSESSMENT?

Depressive disorder, anxiety disorders, and other mental illnesses are typically found with PTSD diagnosis (Doyle & Mitchell, 2003). Case studies have correlated PTSD as a precipitating event of major depressive disorder, complicated grief reaction, schizophrenia, dissociative disorder, and others (Doyle & Mitchell, 2003) for individuals with and without intellectual disorders.

Developmental and intellectual disorders are typically caused by a neurological brain injury. There is a two to three times higher incidence at any point in time of mood disorders associated with developmental and intellectual disabilities (Weisblatt, 2002). This status, coupled with the stress of trauma, seems to precipitate depression in individuals with and without intellectual disabilities.

For individuals with limited language, depression can be observed behaviorally as anxiety, crying spells, fears, sensitivity, deep sadness, and loss of interest in usually gratifying activities. Signs of depression expressed physically can be observed as increased body stress with unexplained nausea, headaches, pains, eating problems, low energy, regressive behaviors, sleep problems, and nightmares (Reiss, 1988). While the common association of depression is a passive, withdrawn state, depression also can appear as irritability, agitation, aggression, and even self-injurious behaviors. The skilled therapist must be aware of the subtle symptoms of trauma and mood disorders. These will help the therapist determine whether or not to seek a psychiatric consultation to evaluate the necessity of medication as an adjunct to treatment. When depression is diagnosed and treated correctly, quickly, and effectively, there is a better overall lifetime response (Weisblatt, 2002).

The effects of antidepressant medications to treat depression and diminish the Fight/Flight/Numb cycle of PTSD can augment treatment. Establishing the therapeutic relationship and teaching self-soothing behaviors can be the focus of therapy while waiting the 2–6 weeks that are typical for antidepressant medications to reach therapeutic levels.

Antidepressant medications help create a soothing state for an individual and enhance the ability of an individual to employ self-soothing behaviors. While medications are not necessary for everyone, they can be invaluable in treatment. In addition to their positive effects, there are also potential negative effects and unfamiliar feelings that an individual may experience when starting an antidepressant medication.

Lanie's physician reviewed the symptoms of depression that Lanie prepared with her therapist. The symptoms included a loss of interest in typically gratifying activities, isolating herself in her room, overall sadness, weight gain, loss of energy, and poor sleep quality with overnight awakenings. Lanie experienced relief from an antidepressant medication. She also began an exercise program, and this physical activity helped stabilize her.

Treatment

Healing is defined as having memories of the abuse events only when one chooses to recall them, rather than having these memories come, uninvited and intrusively; having feelings (associated with the events) that are bearable; and having manageable symptoms (Herman, 1992).

An individual does not need to disclose every detail and incident pertaining to his or her trauma for successful treatment to happen. Rather, the skills the therapist teaches and the individual masters can be used by the individual to improve his or her ability to cope with unwanted and distressing thoughts or feelings that may arise. Traditional expressive talk therapy alone will not produce healing for individuals with intellectual disabilities.

At the beginning of therapy, the therapist should establish a baseline of symptoms and use them to objectively measure progress, especially if the individual is taking an antidepressant medication. Many of the symptoms of PTSD and depression will improve with therapy, increased coping skills, active and passive exercises, and, for some individuals, medication.

The goals of therapy are to stabilize and soothe an individual by employing coping strategies (specific to the individual's preference, both alone or in public), and process the event in order to put it into context. Coping is not a linear process; revisiting and improving on understanding and skills is expected and continues until there is a level of stability and coping strategies are mastered to an optimal degree. It must be understood that the traumatic event remains a part of the individuals' history and the healing process is best described as a method for coping with it.

Therapeutic treatment hours are usually from 45 to 50 minutes long with insightful conversations but for persons with intellectual disabilities dividing the hour into three distinct periods can create a soothing and expected routine. This division allows the therapist to address the attention span and learning needs of the individual. Establishing routines within the treatment hour is soothing and allows the individual to know what to expect. The first segment is a review of the week and perhaps disclosing new material. The second segment is skill building or modifications. The third segment is developing a written or graphic plan for skill building until the next session. The individual and therapist should identify strengths and strategies for the individual to use to cope. The support person needs to recommit to encouraging the individual to use these strategies outside of the therapeutic hour.

While treatment suggestions must be specific to the individual, the person must be given techniques to relax that are both passive and active. One passive relaxation tool is to have the individual sit comfortably in a chair, place his or her two feet on the floor, and repeat, for example, "My name is Lanie. I am 29 years old and I am safe now. I can choose to be happy now." It is helpful to tape this with soothing music in the background and to suggest use of isometric exercises or relaxing images. For soothing activities outside of the treatment hour, bubble baths, hand rubs, and other multisensory activities are also comforting to some individuals as additional passive treatment strategies to control memories and feelings.

Active relaxation might include exploring where tension is held. Individuals can present with many somatic complaints, but tension is often noted as a knot in the stomach. A specific exercise plan, such as brisk walking or dancing, can be an effective active coping strategy to help reduce this tension. Alternative options include crafts, cooking, drawing, or writing in a journal. By redirecting energy to a productive activity, the tension can be reduced so that the individual experiences relief.

Similarly, there are many options a therapist can use to help an individual increase the feeling of safety. The therapist, for example, should help the individual identify a "safe person" that he or she can speak with and confide in if a new experience or other symptoms arise (Walker-Hirsch & Champagne, 1986). The individual also may find it helpful to learn self-talk: repeating a soothing phrase that the individual has chosen to oneself silently or aloud if experiencing distressing memories or distress. The "safe people" in an individual's life can be reassuring of current safety and can repeat the words with the individual while encouraging soothing behaviors.

Abstract Concepts

Lanie's initial presentation elicited guilt, as if she had caused the rapes. This was expressed by her feelings of "being in trouble" and her hesitancy in answering questions. The abuser had told Lanie that it was her fault that he was raping her because she was pretty. He blamed her for his acts and told her that it would be her fault if his wife divorced him or if he lost his job. Lanie's support staff was able to remind her throughout the day and night that the perpetrator was in jail, not her. They reminded her that everyone supporting her knew it was not her fault and they reminded her to use her new coping strategies she learned in therapy.

One of the challenges in therapy is to transform abstract concepts into concrete images to facilitate understanding and healing. Terms such as *guilt, shame,* and *blame* must be made as concrete as possible. The therapist can create behavioral actions to demonstrate the meaning of abstract words. For example, *guilt* means doing something wrong. To help an individual understand that he or she is not guilty or to blame for what has occurred, the following role-play scenario can be used.

Take a cotton ball or other nondangerous material and warn the individual that you are going to do something "bad." Flick the cotton ball off of the table and tell the person that he or she made the therapist do this. Repeat this action as many times as necessary in an overly exaggerated manner, telling the person the words of the perpetrator. Try to blame the person for making you throw the object. Carefully assess the person's response to these actions and continue the object throwing and supposed blame until the absurdity of blaming the individual becomes apparent. Telling a person that it is their fault that the object is being thrown because they are pretty, as with Lanie, (or using other words of the perpetrator) can facilitate understanding that the victim is truly innocent. The individual will understand that the object throwing is clearly the act and blame of the therapist and that this fact has nothing to do with the individual, who has done nothing to cause the "bad behavior" of the therapist.

While guilt is experienced as doing something bad, shame is experienced as if a person is inherently bad and deserving of abuse. Shame contributes to low self-esteem and sadness. Shame contributes to believing that the distress of the abuse experience is a result of an individual's character. People who have a disability often have their self-esteem assaulted in regard to their disability or their sexuality. In a personal conversation, Leslie Walker-Hirsch recounted an incident of a person with an intellectual disability telling others not to listen to a radio host. The person reported that the radio host used the word *retard* and was insulting to everyone with intellectual disabilities. When the individual was asked what that word meant, the individual did not know, but said that the host always said the word in an angry way. This individual was sure the host meant it as a hurtful insult to that individual personally. The individual had even seen the word *retard* written in his own file and so was sure the radio host was talking about him.

Reframing abusive incidents in light of the cotton ball exercise discussed above can be enlightening and can relieve the person greatly. Reminding the individual that the coercion and trickery was overpowering puts the blame squarely on the perpetrator and shame is diminished.

Lanie's therapist told her to look at the therapist and say whether she thought her therapist had ever been a victim of abuse. Lanie guessed yes, then no, and then continued to alternate back and forth, while the therapist maintained a neutral face. Lanie was confused because she could not decide the answer just by looking at her therapist. The therapist used this uncertainty to show that no one could look at her and detect her experiences or know her thoughts. Lanie experienced a great deal of relief when she felt that no one could know about her victimization unless she chose to reveal it. No one could see and judge her or shame her or feel she wore a "scarlet letter." She was better able to blame her abuser and not herself for the abuse that had been perpetrated. She was asked to repeat: "HE did it to ME. It was HIS fault. HE was wrong. I did nothing bad. I am a good person."

The individual also needs to be reminded there have been many good, kind people in his or her life and only this ONE bad perpetrator!

Another useful tool in clarifying blame, shame, and safety is the CIRCLES®[1] concept. This concept outlines six concentric circles surrounding an individual with the individual being the center of the circles and deciding who will be close to them (Champagne and Walker-Hirsch, 1996). The individual learns that he or she is a highly valued, important person who has strengths and talents that are unique. The individual learns that the perpetrator invaded private personal space without permission and committed a crime by violating his or her person and body. The concrete CIRCLES® example clearly defines and labels the boundaries that the individual has the right to control. This allows the individual to actually see that he or she was innocent of wrongdoing. The CIRCLES® paradigm also establishes that there are many more good people who surround the individual, with whom mutually satisfying relationships with varying degrees of intimacy are possible (Champagne & Walker-Hirsch, 1996).

The individual dictates the healing process and the implementation plan. If the individual wants to share a new memory or symptom with his or her support person, the therapist and the individual agree that this information should sometimes be shared with the therapist as well. Also agreed upon are how and when the new skills will be implemented and whether or not a formal or informal monitoring system is needed. The development of the plan with words and pictorial support for language are dictated by the individual's needs or requests and the therapist's suggestions. The support person is asked to assist in carrying out the plan and assures that there is a person available at various sites frequented by the individual during the day and night to implement this therapeutic process wherever it may be needed.

Treatment typically continues for six to twelve sessions. It is imperative that the individual, family, and support personnel understand that treatment does not begin and end in the office; rather, treatment must occur in all environments to meet the individual's needs. On occasion, individuals return to therapy for a brief period of time after a personal milestone, such as beginning a new relationship or by being triggered with unexpected intensity or duration.

---

[1]The registered trademark CIRCLES® and the descriptive materials herein drawn from copyrighted material in The CIRCLES® Series are used with the expressed permission of James Stanfield Company. All rights reserved. Duplication in any form is prohibited. For information about the CIRCLES® Video Series, contact James Stanfield Publishing Company, 800-421-6534, or visit www.stanfield.com.

Teaching decision-making skills, practicing assertiveness skills, and providing language to report suspicious behavior will lessen the chance of abuse. There are no guarantees that abuse will not happen again! This should not be promised, although it is tempting to do so.

Lanie's message is simple but powerful: "When somebody like me shows (by behavioral or affective symptoms) or says I'm being abused, it is your job to believe."

Although sexual abuse is certainly a tragic occurrence, therapy can provide an excellent opportunity for creating strength from adversity; for raising awareness of parents, professionals, and support staff; and for educating others about recognizing the overall vulnerability of individuals with intellectual disabilities. The memories of abuse will always be a part of that individual, but good treatment and support can allow for future relationships that can be mutually satisfying and enhancing.

While healing is a tremendous feat, prevention is by far a greater accomplishment! It often goes unheralded as individuals, their family members, and the professionals and others who care for and about them learn and teach social and sexual awareness, anatomy and physiology, personal boundaries, language for meaningful sexual communication, and assertiveness behaviors every day of every year.

Preventing sexual abuse and providing treatment to those who have been offended against are important steps to increase the likelihood of rich and fulfilling lives for individuals with intellectual disabilities.

REFERENCES

American Psychiatric Association. (2000). *Diagnostic and Statistical Manual of Mental Disorders* (4th ed.). Washington, DC: Author.

Champagne, M., & Walker-Hirsch, L. (1996). *CIRCLES: Intimacy and Relationships.* Santa Barbara, CA: James Stanfield Co.

Doyle, C., & Mitchell, D. (2003). Posttraumatic stress disorder and people with learning disabilities: A literature based discussion. *Journal of Learning Disabilities,* 7(1), 22–33.

Herman, J.L. (1992). *Trauma and recovery.* New York: Basic Books.

Johnson, M. (1999). *Criminal thinking distortions.* Paper presented at the 3rd Annual Broken Boundaries Conference, Warwick, RI

Kilpatrick, D. (2004). What is violence against women? Defining and measuring the problem. *Journal of Interpersonal Violence, 19*(11), 1209–1234.

Levitas, A.S., & Gilson, S.F. (2001). Predictable crises in the lives of people with mental retardation. *Mental Health Aspects of Developmental Disabilities, 4*(3), 89–100.

Nettleback, T., Wilson, C., Potter, R., & Perry, C. (2000). The influence of inter-personal competence on personal vulnerability of persons with mental retar-dation. *Journal of Interpersonal Violence, 15*(1), 46–62.

Petersilia, J., Foote, J., & Crowell, N.A. (2001). *Crime victims with developmental dis-abilities: Report of a workshop.* Washington, DC: National Academies Press.

Reiss, S. (1988). *Reiss screen for maladaptive behavior.* Worthington, OH: IDS Pub-lishing Corporation.

Reynolds, L.A. (1997). *People with mental retardation and sexual abuse.* Silver Spring, MD: The Arc Q&A.

Sobsey, D. (1994). *Violence and abuse in the lives of people with disabilities.* Baltimore: Paul H. Brookes Publishing Co.

Stermac, L., & Del Bove, G. (2004). Stranger and acquaintance sexual assault of adult males. *Journal of Interpersonal Violence, 19*(8), 901–915.

Tarasoff v. University of California, No. 7 Cal. 3d 425.

Walker-Hirsch, L. & Champagne, M.P. (1986). *CIRCLES: Stop Abuse.* Santa Bar-bara, CA: James Stanfield Co.

Wall, B.W., Krupp, B.H., & Guilmette, T. (2003). Restoration of competency to stand trial: A training program for persons with mental retardation. *Journal of the American Academy of Psychiatry and the Law, 31,* 189–201.

Weisblatt, S. (2002, June). *Tools for Working with Children and Adults that are Dual-ly Diagnosed.* Paper presented at the National Association of Dually Diagnosed conference, New Windsor, NY.

13

Sexuality and Mental Health

Interventions and Treatment

Robert Joseph and John J. Barisa

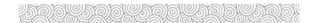

A person with an intellectual disability often has a diminished capacity to understand the generally accepted rules of social interaction and the "unwritten rules" of interaction. This often leads to the fear and anxiety people with intellectual disabilities have when interacting with others, as well as the anxiety people without disabilities may have when interacting with people who have disabilities. The consequence of this fear and anxiety is often that people tend to avoid, either consciously or unconsciously, these interactions. This leaves the person with an intellectual disability either unaware or naive, or undereducated about interactions. This concern applies foremost to social interactions. One can imagine how these interactions become more complicated if a sexual component is involved. When sexual impulses, desire, and feelings are introduced, the understanding of interactions for the person with an intellectual disability becomes increasingly more difficult.

A person often experiences discomfort and/or dysfunction when not able to manage the routines of daily life because his or her sexuality interferes with the ability to function in a supporting environment. Discomfort may include shyness, fear of intimacy, and withdrawal. Dysfunction may include inappropriate sexual behavior, such as public displays of sexual behavior, or force or coercion perpetrated on others. This discomfort and dysfunction may lead to a sexual disorder. When an individual's sexual issues interfere with daily routines of life, he or she may be unable to attain satisfaction, happiness, or contentment in their life. Different degrees of anxiety may appear.

Issues of sexuality can be further complicated for people who have intellectual disabilities due to mental delays associated with varying degrees of mental retardation. Issues of sexuality can also be complicated by multiple disabling conditions that can impede functional and healthy sexuality. This may include motor coordination difficulties, especially with individuals with cerebral palsy. Sexuality can be further complicated by people with intellectual disorders who also have other psychiatric conditions. Psychotropic medications can readily interfere with healthy sexuality. Psychiatric symptoms themselves alter perceptions and may evoke diminished self-control and increased impulsivity.

Individuals may experience a loss of connectedness with others due to their diminished capacity for developing meaningful relationships. Consequences may include rejection, isolation, and stigmatization. A sense of being alone and loneliness may contribute to depression, which may then cause diminished self-control or increased impulsivity.

This chapter seeks to address the myriad of issues that people with intellectual disabilities face when they experience their emerging sexuality and seek to channel it into satisfactory sexual experiences and sexual lives. The course that a person must take to move from sexual concern to satisfaction is initiated with an assessment of his or her strengths and weaknesses in terms of sexuality knowledge and understanding. This assessment directs the treatment that takes the form of sex education, sexuality counseling, behavior management, and/or sex therapy.

ASSESSMENT

The most important component associated with the understanding and treatment of sexuality and sexual issues with people with intellectual disabilities or other mental health issues is a clear and extensive sexuality assessment administered by a trained psychologist or social worker. A thorough assessment seeks to uncover an individual's knowledge and understanding of sexuality and sexual behavior. This would include inquiry specifically concerning relationships, sexual contact, consent, birth control, sexually transmitted diseases, and self-protection. Some people lack good knowledge and understanding. This is distinguished from those who have reasonable understanding but choose to act in ways that violate reasonable parameters for social and sexual interaction. Assessments must include how issues in sexuality interfere with daily routines and activities. Assessments should have a clear understanding of the individual's current sexual thoughts, emotions, and behaviors. This will create the structure of any treatment process or procedure. A relevant sexual history of the individual contributes to the assessment. The assessment should include a risk intensity scale of past or predictable behavior patterns of sexual offenses toward others or themselves. The risk intensity scale identifies the sexual behavior of concern, in addition to its frequency and intensity. For example, how often does a person masturbate in public places? Or, how often does a person engage in sexual contact with a person who is not capable of giving consent? People with sexual naiveté or underdevelopment of sexuality are excellent candidates for sexual education and counseling.

Assessments should also include the individual's global abilities in functioning. A clear understanding of the person's strengths, weaknesses, and limitations is essential for deriving a meaningful and compelling treatment plan. Treatments will need to be adapted for individuals with varying cognitive skills and deficits to ensure each individual's learning and growth. The assessment should also assess the danger to self or others and any physical limitations that would interfere with sexual performance.

A thorough assessment must precede any education, counseling, or therapy. It is suggested that key components be included in the assessment. Such components include an individual's present living situation and day program or work involvement, impressions on the person's personality and needs structure, and background information, especially if extenuating circumstances led to the referral for assessment (i.e., predatory behavior or victim of abuse). The assessment should determine the individual's environmental awareness and understanding of emotions, gender and anatomy issues, relationship issues, personal hygiene, public versus private behavior, sexual intercourse and consequences, birth control, sexually transmitted diseases, and social skills.

During an assessment, the therapist should determine whether the individual has the capacity to consent to sexual contact based on state law. As an overview, this capacity would include 1) understanding and being responsible for the potential consequences of sexual contact, 2) understanding privacy as it relates to sexual contact, 3) understanding infection control and safer sex, and 4) understanding personal safety, rights of others, and the ability to communicate with others if help is needed. Clinical observations and impressions would contribute important information to the final determination of an individual's capacity to consent to sexual contact. The assessment concludes with recommendations for education, treatment, and/or protective oversight.

TREATMENT

Treatment strategies and methods for people with intellectual disabilities who present sexuality concerns vary based on the needs of each individual. For individuals who are attending day programs or living in residential facilities, treatment frequently begins with external control, emphasizing supervision, monitoring, and protective oversight to assure the health, safety, and welfare of all involved. The treatment for the presenting sexuality concern is then implemented. Treatment may include sex education, behavior management, counseling, and sex therapy. The goal of treatment is to provide training for healthy sexuality.

The goal of sex education, counseling, and therapy is to enrich individuals' quality of life by assisting them in attaining appropriate expressions of sexuality. Appropriate expressions of sexuality are characterized by a person engaging in sexual contact with another person with consent, free of coercion or force. Inappropriate contact would include touching without permission from the person being touched or using the other person to stimulate one's own genitalia (frotteurism). Appropriate expressions should include satisfying sexual experiences that respect the needs and feelings of others without causing discomfort or exploiting others. Additional goals are to provide individuals with the ability to identify the appropriate time, place, and circumstance for sexual behavior. The objective is to help the individual understand how to express sexuality in an appropriate, safe, and healthy manner.

STRATEGIES FOR EDUCATION AND COUNSELING

People with challenging issues in sexuality should first receive treatment geared toward a clear and thorough understanding of sexuality through a concise sex education curriculum or program. A well-developed sex education program will include education in anatomy, gender differences, hygiene, self-respect, social skills and dating, basic human reproduction and birth control, physical affection and touch, relationships, sexual contact, sexually transmitted disease, personal safety and sex abuse prevention, marriage, and parenthood. The essential emphasis throughout all education and training is the appropriateness of time, place, and circumstance to express sexuality. These topics revolve around the primary sexual behaviors of masturbation and consensual activity between two people. Inherent in sex education is the understanding of emotions, sexual drive, and love. The positive consequences of a mutually satisfying relationship, and the negative consequences of potential loss and hurt, need to be considered continuously. Discussions regarding responsibility also occur, emphasizing safer sex issues, birth control, and respect for others. It is important for individuals to know that sex can harm other people physically as well as emotionally, and that it is important to respect and consider other people's feelings in the process.

Using concrete and visual representation with pictures of situations is often helpful for individuals with intellectual disabilities. The use of illustrated facial expressions of emotions, for example, can enhance the understanding of emotion. Individuals with intellectual disabilities often experience difficulty articulating emotions, feelings, and thoughts. In addition, these same individuals often do not have a vocabulary of sexual terms for assisting them in identifying their feelings and expressing themselves. Thus, interventions should include assisting the patient to connect his or her sexual feelings to sexual actions using a vocabulary that enables the individual to describe and communicate his or her feelings in a meaningful manner.

BEHAVIOR MANAGEMENT

The following case study is an example of a treatment program for sexuality habilitation. This example teaches safe and healthy sexuality. The goal is for the individual to improve his social/sexual behavior patterns. The treatment objective is for the person to display no inappropriate social/sexual behavior within 1 year. Therapeutic training includes reviewing with the person his social roles and boundaries. The therapist and patient develop systems for the patient to understand issues associated with his own personal sexuality. Primarily, the individual needs to understand the distinction between fantasy and reality. The individual needs assistance in understanding that fantasy within sexual thoughts needs to remain within his own thoughts and must not move into reality unless that behavior is within the boundaries that were first established. The individual also needs assistance to understand temptation and how it affects behavior. When temptation increases in intensity and behavior outside the boundaries is considered, the individual needs to know how to access assistance.

Intervention strategies include reviewing with the individual appropriate interactions, social roles, and boundaries. If the individual displays inappropriate autoerotic sexual behaviors, he is to be redirected to the appropriate place and time to express such behavior. If the person engages in inappropriate sexual contact behavior, he is to be redirected to appropriate alternative behaviors of his daily routines or preferred leisure interests and activities. This should redirect his thoughts and emotions. If the individual engages in any inappropriate excitement or verbalizes any suggestion of influence, attention, or advancement, or shows signs of agitation or staring while in the community, he is to be returned to his program/home immediately. Arousal does not redirect easily and it is more effectively addressed in the appropriate place and time. At the first available time after the event was interrupted, the individual must be spoken with about his or her behavior, why it was inappropriate, and what behavior or behaviors would have been reasonable for the person to exhibit. Discussions of the individual's motivation, needs, and emotions would occur depending on the individual's capabilities to understand such issues. An appropriate person to have this discussion with the individual would be a trained professional who knows the individual, such as a psychologist or social worker.

Larry is 35 years old and has mild mental retardation. He possesses a strong sexual drive and seeks relationships with multiple partners. Although Larry understands safer sexual practices, it is unknown and indeterminable if he uses condoms on a regular basis. Larry has a girlfriend who he considers very important to him. However, he has not shown any true commitment or fidelity to her. After sexual contact with other females, Larry experiences substantial guilt. He then seeks to decrease his guilt by admitting to his girlfriend that he had sex with another person. This hurts his girlfriend and he always promises to be "loyal for now on" to make her feel better. This promise, however, creates the false impression that their relationship will be better.

In counseling, Larry has revealed that he "loves sex." The therapist's impression is that Larry will not cease seeking multiple partners without a behavior management plan in place in addition to counseling.

The behavior management plan is devised with Larry in his counseling session. In addition, staff persons from Larry's supported community living apartment are invited to participate, as they spend significant time together and will thus enhance the oversight of the behavior management plan.

Larry's behavior management plan includes 1) awareness, 2) education, and 3) reinforcement of positive behavior. Awareness for Larry focused on risks that he incurs when he does not practice safer sex. Larry recently needed to have a blood test after having unprotected sex in a pay-for-sex situation. He experienced a serious scare that lingers in him. The therapist periodically reminds Larry of this difficult experience. The education component focuses on responsibility, health and safety, and fidelity in his relationship. As a consequence of seeking sex as his highest priority, Larry has a severe deficiency in his repertoire of leisure activities other than sex. The therapist has introduced Larry to alternative activities such as bicycle riding and photography. Larry is encouraged to experience and understand the pleasures available in nonsexual activities. Larry receives praise whenever he engages in and reports on these activities.

Associated with verbal praise for these activities is a cuing system that serves to remind Larry of the availability of these activities. Simple phrases are used to remind Larry of his goals and possible negative consequences of the behavior he is seeking to eliminate. The therapist often reminds Larry to "Keep your eye on the prize" or "Use brain power." These phrases remind Larry of the activities he should pursue if he wants to have a better relationship with his girlfriend. These phrases help him avoid sexual contacts that result in guilt, shame, and anxiety, and which ultimately damage his relationship with his girlfriend. Larry and his therapist devise, explain, discuss, and practice each of these cues throughout each counseling session. When Larry engages in a behavior he wishes to increase, his therapist uses the phrases that commend him and reinforce the behavior. When Larry engages in behaviors he wants to eliminate, his therapist uses phrases that suggest and remind him of negative consequences.

Behavior management has been successful for Larry, as he now has a clearer understanding of the behaviors that he wants to eliminate and what he needs to do to replace those behaviors. Larry has attained a more monogamous and committed relationship with his girlfriend and has enjoyed the secondary gain of pleasure, freedom from guilt, and self-satisfaction.

BEHAVIOR MANAGEMENT AND THE SEX KIT

Residential agencies for people with intellectual disabilities have used a "sex kit" to enhance the teaching of sex education and to help the individual manage their sexual needs. A sex kit can be gathered in a shoe-box-like container and holds items that assist and remind the owner of his sexual behavior and how to engage in it safely. The kit teaches the appropriate time, place, and circumstance to express sexuality. For example, illustrations of areas in which masturbation is allowed and not allowed are often included (e.g., bathroom, allowed; family room, not allowed). The kit includes items tailored to meet the unique needs of the individual and can be stored in his or her bedroom. Such items can include, but are not limited to, lubricant gels, tissues, picture of hygiene upon completion, and, for certain individuals, visual aids and pictures that can help increase arousal. Assistive devices that stimulate the genitalia (e.g., vibrators) may also be included. The kit is a tangible and discreet object that can help to remind a person of safe and healthy sexuality.

The following case study is an example of a treatment program for sexuality habilitation using a sex kit. The treatment objective is that the patient will use the kit at appropriate times and will not engage in any inappropriate sexual behavior. Training procedures entail teaching the person the appropriate use for each item in the kit. In residential settings, this training should occur in the bedroom. Topics to be discussed are appropriateness of time and place. Also to be taught is the descriptive cue that the kit serves. Staff should reinforce the meaning of the kit as a cue for redirection. It is important for the person to learn that the kit is kept in the designated area in the bedroom. It should stay in the bedroom discreetly but visible as a reminder of appropriate sexual behaviors.

Applied training includes the person using the kit. Staff must acknowledge the appropriateness of the person asking to use the kit. Then, staff should give the person the private time desired. If the person seeks to use the kit at inappropriate times, he is redirected back to the activity he is supposed to be engaging in at that particular time. Explain to the person that this is not an appropriate time or place and explain what are the better times and places for using the kit.

Bob is 38 years old and has moderate mental retardation and severe communication difficulties. He has difficulty understanding what people say to him, and he has difficulty expressing his own thoughts and feelings. Bob lives in a group home, and he enjoys masturbation. However, Bob has a history of masturbating in inappropriate places at inappropriate times. He has masturbated in his day program and in public where others may see him. Bob has been nonresponsive to verbal counseling. Bob was an excellent candidate for a sex kit.

For his kit, Bob was given an erotic poster of a naked woman. He had shown great interest in the poster and finds it sexually arousing. Bob's kit also included gel for lubrication, tissues for cleanup, and an illustration of a sink to remind Bob to wash his hands afterwards. Bob learned that when he felt sexually aroused and wanted to masturbate, he needed to get his kit. The staff at his group home helped Bob to find a place in his bedroom to keep his kit. Bob and his therapist agreed that Bob should only masturbate with the kit, a simple association he was able to make and understand.

Previously, Bob had a tendency to announce when he wanted to masturbate by using a crude expression such as "I'm going to jerk off now." Bob was naive, as he did not know any other ways to express himself. Bob's therapist taught Bob expressions that are more acceptable, such as, "can I use my kit now," or "I need to use my kit now."

Bob learned that he needed to masturbate only with his kit, which was kept in his bedroom. Bob valued the sex kit as his own possession. The pleasure he received in association with the kit further enhanced his willingness to masturbate only where the kit was placed. At times Bob would ask the staff if he could go use his kit.

The sex kit was successful for Bob partly because the onset of his sexual arousal had previously been a random occurrence and he found this very confusing. Bob understood that he could masturbate and that he enjoyed it. However, he did not understand the rules concerning appropriate times and places to masturbate. Bob's sex kit provided him with the cues that helped him know "where" and "when" it was okay to masturbate. An added bene-fit of the kit was that staff, especially during the early stage of introducing the kit, were able to become more familiar with the cues that Bob would give when becoming sexually aroused. In the past, he would begin to fondle him-self. Now, staff members are able to intervene by asking Bob, "Where is your kit?" Bob understands what that means and is able to stop himself and go to his kit. Bob is able to do this without feeling that he is being forced to stop and without becoming disturbed, distressed, and/or angered.

SOCIO-SEXUAL COMPONENT

An inherent component of all sexuality education, training, and coun-seling is the social aspect of living in a community and interacting with others. Staff can teach this daily when they model appropriate social behaviors. When staff members interact with other people, they should be aware that the individuals in their care are present and watching. Staff members should model appropriate interactions within appropri-ate boundaries. During the interaction, staff may include the person in the social situation and teach the appropriateness of greeting, shaking hands, maintaining a social conversation, and departure behavior. Once the applied lessons are complete and the social situation has ended, staff members should briefly process with the person how well, or not, the sit-uation went. Compliment appropriate behaviors and teach alternative behaviors for inappropriateness.

It is important to provide these therapies and training proactively each day, especially when the person receiving treatment is calm and functioning relatively well. The therapist and individual should practice these techniques with demonstration and repetition.

The therapist may focus on specific behaviors during training and education. For example, what functions are served when hugging or kiss-ing another person? There exist important distinctions between social or familial hugging and kissing and romantic hugging and kissing. Also, where are the places in which it is okay to engage in romantic or sexual interactions? Is it okay to engage in sexual touching if no one is there to see, even though it may not take place in a private place (i.e., sexual con-tact allowed if no one is around in a public park)?

Michelle is 26 years old and has severe mental retardation and Down syn-drome. Michelle lives in a group home. She is very friendly and enjoys the attention of staff and peers. Although Michelle's expressive language skills are very limited, she is able to communicate using one-word phrases and physical gestures. Michelle has a strong sexual drive, as she masturbates regularly, and enjoys physical contact that includes genital stimulation. To attain genital stimulation, Michelle frequently tries to rub her body against others. She does this for sexual arousal and will do it to anyone who responds positively to her request for a hug.

Michelle asks for a hug and gestures toward others with her arms open and a huge smile on her face. People tend to like Michelle and find it to be enjoyable to respond to her requests for a hug. Thus, they become unwitting participants in her sexual behavior. Michelle is in violation of a reasonable boundary as she is engaging in inappropriate sexual contact and doing so without the knowledge or consent of the other person. Michelle not only seeks sexual contact with staff and peers of similar intelligence to her, but she also attempts sexual interactions with lower intellectually functioning people who are unaware of what she is doing to them.

Michelle's social interaction had become inappropriate sexual contact. This concern was addressed in counseling through the use of illustrations, drawings, and role play. However, during the course of Michelle's daily activities, staff members were directed to provide the "socio-sexual" component of treatment. That is, whenever Michelle initiated contact with another person, staff would observe for appropriate greeting behavior. If Michelle attempted to hug the person, staff would lightly remind Michelle that a hello or handshake was "good enough." In that Michelle was aware of what she was not supposed to do, she willingly redirected herself. At the end of the usually brief episode, staff would have Michelle practice appropriate greetings without hugging. They would remind her that excessive hugging and rubbing her body against another person was not allowed. If Michelle demonstrated an appropriate greeting, she received verbal praise and this reinforced her behavior. If Michelle's behavior was inappropriate, staff would emphasize how and why her behavior was inappropriate and how she should have behaved. The staff modeled both appropriate and inappropriate behavior and connected praise or corrective statements to the behavior, such as "that is not right; do not hug like that; say hello like this."

Treatment was successful for Michelle, as she learned which behaviors were inappropriate and restricted, and also which behaviors constituted appropriate interactions. Michelle's sexual needs and behavior were refocused on private areas in her group home. The therapist emphasized that sexual behavior is only for times when she was by herself. Michelle's sexual behavior must be limited to autoerotic activities because she does not have the capacity to consent to sexual contact.

SEXUALITY COUNSELING

Individuals with intellectual disabilities desire the same things in life as all people do; to like and be liked, to love and be loved, and to have meaning in their lives. Sexuality provides an individual with the ability to experience pleasure and meaning. This may take the form of autoerotic or sexual contact pleasure. Individuals often engage in masturbation, as it can provide arousal, stimulation, satisfaction, and relief. Couples can engage in sexual contact for similar reasons and for the connection it creates between two people who care for each other and desire to give pleasure to each other. Sexual contact between two people requires that they both have the capacity to consent to sexual contact and have willingly chosen to have sex with each other.

Individuals with intellectual disabilities often suffer because others want to deny them their right to attain knowledge and understanding about their bodies and their sexuality. The history of sex education in school systems has been fraught with resistance from various groups who reject the notion that young people provided with good information will use it appropriately to protect themselves and others. Rather, it is believed that young people will use information to act indiscriminately, irresponsibly, and destructively. A more insidious belief is that people will not concern themselves about sex if they are not told about it.

Special education programs often have inadequate or nonexistent sex education classes. Often people who are mentally retarded are seen as incapable of understanding sexuality or sexual behavior. Thus, for their "own protection" they are denied the important lessons that others falsely believe will trigger desires and needs. Extrapolated further, people with mental retardation who know about sex will be unable to satisfy their needs and urges, and if they attempt to, society will be placed at risk. Ultimately, people with mental retardation are left unaware and unknowing of sexuality, and they are unable to attend to the desires and needs they feel. These desires and needs may remain unarticulated and misunderstood. Regardless, but understandably, attempts are made to satisfy sexual desires and needs, often with poor outcomes because of the lack of knowledge, not because of the knowledge. Frustration, anger, confusion, and depression may all result. Sexuality counseling seeks to assist the individual to identify these needs, understand them, and safely satisfy them within the reasonable criteria set by one's community and society.

The basic premise of sexuality counseling is to increase a person's ability to identify sexual feelings that he or she is having and to be able to apply a vocabulary to those feelings. Sexuality counseling also needs to identify the behaviors the individual can engage in to express those feelings. Often these sexual feelings are self-directed and the person is able to provide oneself with sexual pleasure. Other times, sexual contact is the focus of counseling. The individual learns to see how to negotiate sexual contact in a relationship and how it represents expressions of interest, desire, affection, and love. Sexuality counseling seeks to help the individual understand the parameters that exist around sexual behavior to determine when sexual behavior is appropriate and mutually and consensually agreed upon, as well as when it is inappropriate or unwanted.

CASE STUDIES

The following case studies are presented to highlight the dilemma that befalls individuals who have developed with a significant void in their life: a lack of sex education and training.

Alan is 35 years old and has mild mental retardation. He was referred for sexuality counseling after he had been discovered masturbating in a public restroom in a bowling alley. Alan revealed that he frequently masturbates in public restrooms of restaurants, bowling alleys, and work program sites. Alan lives in a group home. Informal attempts by staff to dissuade him from engaging in such behavior were not successful. Although Alan agreed that he should not masturbate in public, he apparently continued to do so as he was discovered at various times. Alan's expressed desire to cease was simply his way to evade dealing with staff.

Alan works in a sheltered workshop and attends an evening recreation program. He travels independently throughout his community. Alan often becomes sexually aroused during his travels, which triggers his interest in masturbating. He does not understand the concept of delayed gratification. Rather, he seeks a place in which he can masturbate immediately.

Alan's treatment has focused on cognitive, behavioral, and self-image areas. The therapist started by asking Alan about the thoughts he has while walking in the community. Alan initially responded that he does not think of anything. The therapist began offering ideas of what Alan might be thinking and what other people sometimes think about sexually. The therapist's statements allowed Alan to consider that having sexual thoughts was okay because other people have similar thoughts and that sexual thoughts can appear at anytime during the day. In effect, the therapist allowed Alan to reveal that he looks at women's breasts and that he imagines touching their breasts. Alan talked about getting "excited, having that feeling" and "getting hard." Alan then explained how he "wants to find a restroom to have the white stuff come out." The therapist explored whether Alan felt he could distract himself in order to stop the erection. Alan felt that he could not.

When sexually aroused Alan will enter a public restroom stall and masturbate to orgasm. Alan believes that the stall meets the requirement for privacy. He does not understand that this is not "true" privacy as he would have in his home. Alan does not consider that there are open areas between the slots of the door and walls in which others may see him masturbate. In addition, Alan makes vocal sounds associated with masturbation that are easily heard.

The therapist helped Alan identify the images and thoughts that he finds sexually arousing during his travels. Alan became more aware of his early stages of arousal. The therapist suggested alternative ways to travel without becoming sexually aroused. One way was for the therapist to help Alan map out his trip from place to place in order to avoid wandering. Wandering contributes to observing women and then experiencing arousal and fantasy. Without observation, the progression to arousal and fantasy is disrupted. Alan is asked to concentrate on his destination and to adhere to certain rules of traveling that ensure a quick arrival at the destination.

The therapist also asked Alan to think of behaviors that he can exhibit if he were to begin looking at women and having sexual thoughts. Alan and the therapist devised behaviors such as immediately crossing the street to walk on the other side of the road, or thinking of what he would like to eat for his next meal, or thinking of an interest in sports that he has. The therapist and Alan formulated strategies for disrupting the course of events from observation to fantasy to arousal to searching for a place to masturbate.

Alan and the therapist also worked on increasing his understanding of delayed gratification. Alan underestimates the amount of pleasure he can attain by only engaging in masturbation in the privacy of his home. This includes the pleasures of assistive devices he may use to stimulate arousal such as erotic magazines and videos. In addition, Alan is reminded that he can fall asleep after orgasm only when he is in his own bed. Alan found that he enjoys this. Alan's therapist asked him during counseling to discuss his entire masturbation experience. This allowed Alan to feel comfortable talking about what he had always been told not to talk about because it is private, even secret. Alan has become more accepting of discussing masturbation because he is being asked his thoughts and feelings, not being spoken to or punished. The therapist is highly supportive of masturbation that meets the acceptable criteria of proper time and place. For masturbation that does not, the therapist consistently asks Alan to consider the mistakes that is he making.

Alan has also revealed that he experiences shame and guilt after masturbating. The second cognitive factor in therapy is the use of this shame and guilt to discourage inappropriate masturbation, and to begin the process of resolving these feelings after appropriate masturbation. The therapist has worked on the time factor of the onset of shame and guilt. The therapist seeks to move these feelings closer in time to the onset of searching for a public restroom in which to masturbate. It would benefit Alan to have these feelings at that time in order to disrupt the process. The objective is for Alan to use these feelings as part of his rejection of masturbating in public restrooms. Although the reasons for Alan's shame and guilt may be many and complex, the therapist uses these feelings in a specific way to address a specific need. The therapist seeks to attach these "negative" feelings directly to masturbating in a public restroom. The therapist often asks Alan to talk about how bad he feels about everything related to masturbating in a public restroom. On the other hand, the therapist just as often asks Alan to speak about everything that is positive related to masturbating when in his bedroom.

Lastly, counseling has addressed Alan's self-image issues. Alan expressed that he does not want to be the type of person who is unable to control himself. Alan and the therapist identify episodes in which he resists public restroom masturbation as times in which he successfully met his objective and feels very good about himself. All episodes of self-control are identified and contribute to Alan's positive self-image. Alan is asked to identify positive things in his life. The therapist reacts to each by stating how this shows him to be "a mature person in control of his life." The therapist emphasizes appropriate masturbation as a "positive thing; you are in control," and inappropriate masturbation as a "negative thing; you are not in control." The therapist helps Alan to better understand the connections between his behavior and what he thinks about himself, by attaching positive self-statements to positive behaviors and negative self-statements to negative behaviors.

Alan has significantly decreased his frequency of inappropriate masturbation. However, when his daily activities are less structured, he still struggles with the impulse to masturbate immediately after arousal. When Alan wanders he is more prone to look at females with sexual thoughts and fantasies. Therapy is now focused on the choices he makes when traveling in the community. The fundamental choice that is constantly raised by the therapist is whether he wants to seek a place to masturbate or to suppress his thoughts and feelings until he arrives home where he may masturbate in the appropriate place.

Marvin is 55 years old and has mild mental retardation. He lives in a community residence. Marvin was referred for sexuality counseling as he has engaged in sexually provocative behavior. He secretly tries to fondle his genitalia on the top of his pants while in conversation with females. In addition, Marvin engages in a range of sexually inappropriate behaviors, such as singing songs with altered lyrics to include sexually explicit words and acts, urinating in the residence bathroom with the door open, and masturbating in bed under his blanket while asking female staff to come into his room.

Treatment explored Marvin's knowledge and understanding of boundaries. Marvin had an awareness of privacy but a confused sense of what constituted full privacy across various situations. Marvin considered his singing to be private. He did not recognize that his singing was overheard by others and that the content, although humorous to him, may not be similarly perceived by others. Marvin explained, "I sing to myself under my breath."

Marvin believed that masturbation in his bedroom was private in that he only did it where he was told was the appropriate place. When he asked a female staff member to come into his room to rearrange something, he continued to believe that he was masturbating in private because his genitalia were covered. He explained, "my penis was under the blanket; she couldn't see it." Marvin was singularly focused on one aspect of privacy rather than the context in which it occurred.

Marvin needed to increase his understanding of privacy across various situations and contexts. The therapist asked Marvin to identify the meaning of privacy. Marvin responded, "in my bed." Marvin's explanation did not sufficiently include the larger context in which it takes place. The therapist explained that although the bedroom is considered a private room it does not remain private if there is another person in the bedroom. Primarily, Marvin did not understand the need to be alone as the necessary component of privacy rather than just being in a private place. Marvin was continuously asked to make distinctions between private behaviors and private places.

Treatment then addressed the arousal component of Marvin's sexual behaviors. Marvin possesses a strong sexual drive. He frequently acted indiscriminately on his sexual feelings. This led to singing, self-fondling, and asking others suggestive questions (e.g., inquiring if a female staff member would be having sex with her husband that evening). Marvin did this to increase his sexual arousal and contribute to his sexual pleasure. Marvin did not sufficiently assess the consent or willingness of the other person to be part of his sexual behavior. Marvin needed to understand that this was coercive, deceptive, and inappropriate. Essentially, Marvin believed that if the object of his sexual interest was unaware of his intent or behavior, then it would *not* be inappropriate. The therapist asked Marvin to consider how his actions may make the other person feel if they were aware of what he was doing. Immediately after each comment that Marvin made about his behavior he was asked to place himself "in the other person's shoes" and to consider what she may be seeing and thinking and feeling. After each successful exercise in which Marvin stated that the other person might be annoyed, angered, disgusted, upset, and so forth, the therapist asked Marvin to consider what that says about himself. The objective was to have Marvin understand his effect on others by imagining himself as the other. Treatment is considered more and more successful as Marvin increases his ability for empathy and to control his behavior as he understands the negative effect it can have on others.

Elizabeth is 28 years old with mild mental retardation who lives in a supported apartment. She was referred for sexuality counseling because she was engaging in public sexual contact. Elizabeth had been assessed and determined to have the capacity to consent to sexual contact. Thus, she was free to exercise her right to visitation and privacy in her supported apartment. Elizabeth and her boyfriend, John, were discovered engaging in sexual intercourse in the alley behind their workshop building. They were immediately asked to cease and dress as their contact was inappropriate in terms of place and time. They were upset and embarrassed, and the workshop director spoke with each of them about their actions.

Elizabeth was resistant to reveal that she was having sex. It is likely that she had learned that it was better to deny having had sex, or to lie altogether, than to tell the truth as she had been admonished for having sex in the past. Unfortunately, this behavior resulted in allegations being made against a partner in spite of the sex being mutually consensual. People with intellectual disabilities are often fearful that they will get into trouble and be punished for behaving sexually.

The staff for Elizabeth's supported apartment work in an office in the same apartment building. There is much interaction between Elizabeth and the staff.

Sexuality counseling focused on Elizabeth's behavior. She first explained that she and John are "boyfriend and girlfriend." Elizabeth chose to have sex in the alley because she believed that she would "get into trouble" if she brought John into her apartment for sex. Elizabeth was fully aware that the alley was a poor choice of place for sexual contact, and she was sufficiently aware of the danger involved in public sexual contact. It is important to note that people with intellectual disabilities tend not to articulate their feelings and thoughts very clearly. In this case, Elizabeth made statements such as "I know it's bad, I know it's wrong, I could get hurt." The therapist understood "could get hurt" to mean that another person could come upon her and John and possibly take advantage of, or hurt, them. The therapist determined that Elizabeth had expressed the ability to adequately assess the risks and rewards of public sexual contact and apparently had done so. Elizabeth stated, "I did it anyway because I thought I could get away with it."

Elizabeth's supported apartment program is committed to protecting her right to visitation and privacy. However, Elizabeth's lack of knowledge led her to be afraid to ask for permission to have John in her apartment. She believed that she would be chastised for wanting to have sex and that it was "against the rules."

Ongoing sexuality counseling focused on Elizabeth's understanding of her rights and responsibilities. The therapist explained to Elizabeth how she is a person like her peers, her siblings, and other people she knows who likely have sex also. The patient often believes that opportunities for intimacy, romance, love, and sex are only for other people. The patient may not feel entitled to have such feelings, no less, to engage in sex. To allay Elizabeth's anxieties about how staff may react to her request for privacy, counseling helped her formulate what she might say to staff when she wanted to inform them that she would be bringing a guest to her apartment. It is essential to note that in accordance with Elizabeth exercising her right to privacy and visitation she would be informing staff, not asking permission.

Therapy was successful as Elizabeth has effectively developed the skill to inform staff that she is bringing a guest into the apartment. Elizabeth understands that it is not their job to say "no," but rather, they are concerned about her social life and want to support her. Elizabeth feels closer to trusted staff members as she feels that they listen to her. For Elizabeth, this means that they understand and respect her interest in sex and desire for a "real boyfriend." Elizabeth now feels entitled to have these feelings and to act on them.

Iris is 45 years old with mild mental retardation. Walter is 52 years old with borderline intelligence and a history of verbal hostility and depression. They have been together for 18 years and have lived together for the past 10 years. Iris and Walter were referred for sexuality counseling as they expressed the desire to increase their intimate sexual contact. Iris and Walter entered counseling as a couple in distress. They argued constantly, and their conversation style was problematic. Walter would interrupt Iris as soon as she spoke, and Iris would turn away and make faces when Walter spoke. Walter frequently threatened to leave home and end their relationship. Iris was anxious and fearful, paralyzed to express her feelings or to engage in reasonable conversation to address their problems. Walter was angry and hostile; Iris was passive and mute.

The therapist started by stating that their counseling sessions would provide each of them the opportunity to speak without disruption. The therapist also stated that he would protect both Iris and Walter from being attacked by the other or ignored. The therapist offered safety and asked for trust.

Early sessions with Iris and Walter provided the therapist with ample opportunity to show that he will stop the hostility, restrict any disruption, and allow each person to fully make his or her point. The therapist was able to gain trust as he made good on his promise not to allow hostility, overt or subtle, to take place in session. The therapist needed to remind Iris and Walter that they could try this at home but he cautioned that it was unlikely they would succeed without a lot of practice in their counseling sessions. The therapist wanted to guard against unrealistic expectations and consequent disappointment. The therapist made the observation that he was acting "like a traffic cop." The therapist occasionally used sweeping motions with his arms to signal one person to continue talking and the other to stop. This injected some levity to ease the tension, but it was also effective in allowing each to speak while the other was directed to listen. Iris and Walter would each speak only to the therapist. The therapist occasionally asked the partner to comment.

On occasion Walter attempted to control the conversation and intimidate Iris. This was forbidden as he was directed to only express himself without being threatening. In a different manner but as damaging to counseling, Iris would become anxious and withdrawn. These episodes required direct emotional support from the therapist and the guarantee that she was in a safe place in which she was free to speak.

Walter was disappointed and angry that they did not have sex as frequently as he desired. Walter was reluctant to express this to Iris as he feared that she would label him a "sex fiend." The therapist asked Walter to talk freely about his sexual desires. He needed to be helped to avoid making direct references to ex-girlfriends as this bothered Iris. Walter was asked to explain why he desires sex with Iris. Walter expressed various feelings about sex. He enjoyed the physical pleasure and the closeness he would feel toward Iris. He feels that sex is normalizing for him. Walter felt as if he was like "other people" because he had sex. Walter never explained these feelings to Iris. Iris would also short-circuit any attempt he did make to tell her his feelings. She did this as self-protection because she immediately believed he was about to criticize her and threaten to leave. In reality, Walter only threatened to leave after she refused to allow him to tell her his feelings. The therapist helped Walter explain the reasons he wanted to have sex. Because the therapist would not allow Iris to turn away and ignore Walter, she was able to hear and acknowledge what he was saying. Iris heard expressions of caring and interest that she had never heard before. She was flattered, warmed, nurtured, and very importantly, sexually aroused.

Iris felt that their relationship problems overwhelmed any desire she may have had for sex. She was also fearful of sexual contact, as she felt that she lacked the skill necessary due to her limited experience. Iris was anxious revealing her concerns about sex, especially with Walter, who often threatened to leave her over the same issue.

In spite of their problems, Iris and Walter's relationship did include mutual caring, respect, and love. It was important for the therapist to use these feelings to construct a foundation for them to be willing to discuss their problems. This therapist frequently underscored their statements with comments about their long-term feelings for each other. This was particularly important as Iris and Walter's cognitive deficits made it difficult for them to see the objectives of counseling beyond the immediacy of their discord. In effect, counseling served as a reminder of why they wanted to reconcile their relationship in spite of the pain, anxiety, and disappointment they were experiencing during counseling.

Iris and Walter were each asked to express their wishes and desires. Walter expressed that he wanted to be closer physically and emotionally with Iris. Iris had perceived his requests for sex solely as his desire for her to service him for physical pleasure. Her inclination was not to think of sex contact as an expression of love and commitment. Iris expressed her fear of not being able to sexually satisfy Walter because of her lack of skill and experience. Walter had not considered her feelings before as he only heard rejection of him.

The second stage of counseling had Iris and Walter going home with assignments. They were directed to set aside time, which was referred to as "private time," in which they would seek to satisfy a need that they each identified in session. For Iris, sessions focused on her need for Walter to cease threatening to leave and for them to engage in activities that would help her become comfortable about having sex. For Walter, sessions focused on him explaining to Iris what type of touch he finds warm, arousing, and pleasurable, and why it was important for him to experience this with her. Each step included reinforcement, praise, and support from each person to the other.

Iris and Walter started each session with a report on how they experienced their "private time," with feelings and thoughts. Private time became their forum for satisfying each other's needs and to improve their communication about what each one wanted in their relationship. Counseling was deemed successful as it eliminated misconceived notions of the other person's intentions and increased each person's ability to satisfy their partner's needs and desires. Iris and Walter's relationship improved significantly.

OVERVIEW OF CASE STUDIES

The key to sexuality counseling is to help the individual attain the sexual awareness, knowledge, and intelligence that meets his or her need for understanding the role that sex plays in the individual's life. The individual is capable of finding pleasure in sexual activities. He or she needs to know how to experience sexual arousal, how to attain stimulation and satisfaction, and how to do so without violating accepted and reasonable social restrictions on sexual behavior. Fundamentally, that would be the need for privacy for either autoerotic activities or sexual contact between two people if they both have the capacity to consent to sexual contact. All people are capable of learning how to increase sexual stimulation, increase sexual arousal, and have a more satisfying sexual experience.

SEX THERAPY

Some individuals may require sex therapy in order to learn appropriate and healthy sexuality. Sex therapy is more application focused. Sex therapy is a direct approach, using specific methods and techniques by a sex therapist. The goal is to provide treatment to enhance more adaptive ways to express sexuality in a safe and healthy manner. This may be physical or emotional. Sex therapy has different degrees of demonstration and therapeutic applications during treatment. Sex therapy is provided to individuals in order to treat and reduce physical and emotional pain and discomfort during sexual expression and performance. Sex therapy demonstrates specific techniques on how to experience and complete sexual expression to satisfaction and to improve one's quality of life. Sex therapy helps individuals learn how to achieve orgasm and understand the resolution phase. It then demonstrates how to move on and redirect themselves to alternative activity to further enhance their quality of life.

Sex therapy is applied to special populations and person's with special needs by helping them access and adapt their limitations to achieve and complete sexual satisfaction. There is use of adaptive equipment, suggested changes in tactile stimulation, and lessons on how to position oneself for optimal sexual success. Sex therapy always occurs in an appropriate manner within a safe and therapeutic environment.

Sex therapy should only be provided by an experienced and supervised professional. Only specific people would be considered appropriate candidates for such sex therapy and treatment. Human rights committees should be thoroughly informed of the patient's needs, strengths, weaknesses, limitations, specific treatment goals, clinical justification, prognosis, potential complications, and possible side effects. People who "need to know" should be kept informed of the progress on a routine basis. Those who "need to know" would include the staff involved in the patient's concern and their respective supervisors.

Sex therapy can use anatomical props to demonstrate specific techniques and teach the person safer methods at achieving an optimal and satisfactory response. Other techniques can include visual or verbal reminders to stay on task for people with poor attending skills. In order to safeguard against confusion of social roles and their boundaries, the sex therapist should not be a person who has any other role in the patient's life.

Sex therapy represents the most involved level of treatment. Thus, the case of Jack and Louise will be reviewed only briefly to give the reader an idea of the complexity involved.

Jack is 55 years old with average intelligence and cerebral palsy. He has very limited movement below his neck. He uses a motorized wheelchair. His wife, Louise, is 48 years old, also with average intelligence and cerebral palsy. Louise's physical disability is as severe as Jack's but different. Louise experiences the uncontrolled movements of spastic-type cerebral palsy. She needs to be pushed in her wheelchair by an aide. Jack and Louise each require assistance to complete activities of daily living, including undressing and getting into bed. Jack and Louise have been married for 10 years.

Jack and Louise requested sex therapy because they have been unable to find a satisfying position for successful sexual intercourse. The missionary position was too difficult, as Louise was unable to tolerate Jack lying on top of her. Their respective physical disabilities made it impossible for them to try positions that required weight bearing by either person. Unfortunately, their sexual frustration was creating discord in their marriage.

The dual concerns of lack of sexual experience and physical disability were prepotent in therapy. Jack and Louise believed that good sex comes naturally in a marriage. They had difficulty understanding and expressing their frustration and disappointment that this was not necessarily true. Their lack of experience with sexual contact left them believing that, the "man on top position" was the way they "were supposed to do it." It had once been suggested by a friend that they should watch erotic videos to see how they can have intercourse. The acrobatic sex depicted in the videos they watched contributed to their increasing frustration and fear that they would never be able to have sexual intercourse. Lastly, their physical disabilities were experienced as true and permanent obstacles. Consequently, damage to their self-image and self-esteem began to occur along with emerging depression.

The therapist developed a three-pronged treatment approach. First, Jack and Louise needed help to begin to articulate their sexual feelings and desires in graphic and sexually explicit terms. Although they were embarrassed using such terms for the first time, they became acclimated to it within the accepting and encouraging atmosphere of counseling. They came to feel that they were learning a new skill with a new language. Secondly, the therapist introduced various non-weight bearing positions for sexual intercourse. The most popular position for Jack and Louise was the so-called "spooning" position. Drawings, pictures, and pantomime were used to illustrate and demonstrate the position. Thirdly, the therapist needed to help resolve their body-image, self-image, and self-esteem disturbances. This was key if they would be able to feel comfortable while naked in bed planning, and engaging in, sexual intercourse.

Therapy was considered successful as Jack and Louise became more committed to their desire for improved sexual relations. They now believe that good sex does not come naturally and that sex is a skill like other skills. That is, a skill that a person can get better at with an open mind and a lot of practice

CONCLUSION

By understanding sexuality as unique to each individual, in addition to a thorough and comprehensive assessment, sexual habilitation can occur and be very successful in meeting each person's needs. Sexual habilitation can assist people in reaching their optimal potential and can enrich the quality of their lives. Individual treatment programs should be developed and tailored for each unique person's needs. Emphasis should be placed on knowing the person's needs as well as their prognosis, to direct treatment and to provide supervision required. All treatment approaches and tools are not appropriate for all persons. Treatment is chosen carefully, reflecting the person's strengths and weaknesses.

Health, safety, welfare, and risk assessments should be made routinely. Human rights committees should be kept informed throughout the treatment process.

Sex education and counseling should use repetition, demonstration, practice of task, consistent delivery of training and application, and visual and concrete representation of abstract concepts as well as sequencing of activity. Other training methods can be educational and counseling in order to enhance development and continue the habilitation process. The use of cuing systems, diagrams, concrete objects and kits, and close monitoring and supervision are some of the training tools available to enhance and improve sexual expression, satisfaction, and healthy sexuality.

Sex therapy is reserved for the experienced professional. Sex therapy applies demonstration techniques as the treatment method.

Sexual habilitation offers individuals who are naive in sexual matters, or have an underdeveloped understanding of sexuality, the opportunity to have more enriched lives and to enjoy satisfying relationships.

RECOMMENDED READING

Carling, F. (1962). *And yet we are human.* London: Chatto & Windus.

Crocker, J., & Major, B. (1989). Social stigma and self-esteem: The self-protective properties of stigma. *Psychological Review, 96*(4), 608–630.

Goffman, E. (1963). *Stigma: Notes on the management of spoiled identity.* New York: Simon and Schuster.

Katz, I. (1981). *Stigma: A social psychological analysis.* New Jersey: Lawrence Erlbaum Associates.

Weinberg, N. (1984). Physically disabled people assess the quality of their lives. *Rehabilitation Literature, 45,* 13–15.

Zola, I.K. (1982). *Missing pieces: A chronicle of living with a disability.* Philadelphia: Temple University Press.

Index

Page references to figures and tables are indicated by *f* and *t*, respectively.

Transsexual community, 162; *see also*
    Rainbow Support Group (RSG)
Trauma, *see* Posttraumatic stress
    disorder (PTSD)
Treatment issues, *see* Mental health
    interventions and sexuality;
    OB-GYN care; Sexual abuse
    recovery
Triggers of posttraumatic stress
    disorder (PTSD) symptoms,
    255*f,* 256
Tubal ligation, 239–240

University of California, Tarasoff v., 252

Vaccinations in OB-GYN care, 236
Values and consent, 186–187
Vasectomy, 138

Voluntariness and consent, 186
Vulnerability
    acquiescence to authority and, 89,
        249
    to sexual abuse, 21, 152–153,
        248–249
    sexuality education and, 19–24
    social isolation and, 20, 116, 199
    supports and, 183

Web sites
    Alan Guttmacher Institute, 232
    College of Direct Support, 115
    laws on sexual consent, 82
    Self Advocates Becoming
        Empowered (SABE), 113
    sexual risks when using, 19
Wet dreams, 36–37
Willowbrook State School, 101